# Medicine and Biomedical Sciences in Modern History

Series Editors
Carsten Timmermann
University of Manchester
Manchester, UK

Michael Worboys
University of Manchester
Manchester, UK

The aim of this series is to illuminate the development and impact of medicine and the biomedical sciences in the modern era. The series was founded by the late Professor John Pickstone, and its ambitions reflect his commitment to the integrated study of medicine, science and technology in their contexts. He repeatedly commented that it was a pity that the foundation discipline of the field, for which he popularized the acronym 'HSTM' (History of Science, Technology and Medicine) had been the history of science rather than the history of medicine. His point was that historians of science had too often focused just on scientific ideas and institutions, while historians of medicine always had to consider the understanding, management and meanings of diseases in their socio-economic, cultural, technological and political contexts. In the event, most of the books in the series dealt with medicine and the biomedical sciences, and the changed series title reflects this. However, as the new editors we share Professor Pickstone's enthusiasm for the integrated study of medicine, science and technology, encouraging studies on biomedical science, translational medicine, clinical practice, disease histories, medical technologies, medical specialisms and health policies.

The books in this series will present medicine and biomedical science as crucial features of modern culture, analysing their economic, social and political aspects, while not neglecting their expert content and context. Our authors investigate the uses and consequences of technical knowledge, and how it shaped, and was shaped by, particular economic, social and political structures. In re-launching the Series, we hope to build on its strengths but extend its geographical range beyond Western Europe and North America.

*Medicine and Biomedical Sciences in Modern History* is intended to supply analysis and stimulate debate. All books are based on searching historical study of topics which are important, not least because they cut across conventional academic boundaries. They should appeal not just to historians, nor just to medical practitioners, scientists and engineers, but to all who are interested in the place of medicine and biomedical sciences in modern history.

More information about this series at
http://www.palgrave.com/gp/series/15183

David Durnin

# The Irish Medical Profession and the First World War

palgrave
macmillan

David Durnin
UCD Geary Institute for Public Policy
University College Dublin
Dublin, Ireland

Medicine and Biomedical Sciences in Modern History
ISBN 978-3-030-17958-8        ISBN 978-3-030-17959-5    (eBook)
https://doi.org/10.1007/978-3-030-17959-5

Cover credit: Trinity Mirror/Mirrorpix/Alamy Stock Photo

This Palgrave Macmillan imprint is published by the registered company Springer Nature Switzerland AG
The registered company address is: Gewerbestrasse 11, 6330 Cham, Switzerland

# ACKNOWLEDGEMENTS

This book began as a PhD thesis and I am very grateful to several societies and funding bodies for their financial support, including the Irish Research Council, the Women's History Association of Ireland, the Lord Edward Fitzgerald Memorial Fund Committee and the Society for the Social History of Medicine. I wish to thank my academic supervisor Catherine Cox, University College Dublin, for all her help, sound advice and encouragement. I am also thankful to Erica Charters and William Mulligan who examined the thesis on which this book is based. Their suggestions helped me to prepare the manuscript for publication. I owe a debt of gratitude to all the staff of UCD School of History, particularly those who read sections of this work and expertly advised, including Mary E. Daly, Lindsey Earner-Byrne and Tadhg Ó hAnnracháin. I have benefited greatly from the knowledge and friendship of those at the Centre for the History of Medicine in Ireland, UCD. Stephen Bance, Anne Mac Lellan, Alice Mauger, Ian Miller, Kirsten Mulrennan and Peter Reid provided an atmosphere of collegiality and practical support. I am especially indebted to Fiachra Byrne and Laura Kelly who read large sections of this work and offered critical judgement and invaluable suggestions. Thanks also to those at the UCD Geary Institute for Public Policy, including Emma Barron, Susan Butler and Philip O'Connell, for their patience and support while I completed this book.

This work would not have been possible without the expertise of the staff at various archives and libraries including the National Archives of Ireland, the Royal College of Physicians of Ireland, the National Library of Ireland, the National Archives (Kew), Trinity College Dublin's Manuscript and Archive's Library, the Royal College of Surgeons in Ireland, the Wellcome Trust Library, the Imperial War Museum and the Public Record Office of Northern Ireland. I am especially grateful to Brian Donnelly (NAI) and Harriet Wheelock (RCPI) for being generous with their time and advice. Sincere thanks also to the team at Palgrave Macmillan, especially Molly Beck and Maeve Sinnott, for their professionalism and guidance through the publication process. Many thanks also to the series editors and the anonymous reviewers for their invaluable comments.

Finally, I would like to thank all my friends and family for their support. A special thanks to my sisters Maria and Molly who continue to inspire in their own pursuits. Thank you to my parents, Mary and Paul. Their support, advice, constant encouragement and above all, their friendship, are of the utmost importance to me. Finally, Carol Faulkner has lived with this work for too many years. She has shown an extraordinary level of patience and understanding. Without her love and guidance, I could not have finished it. In a completely inadequate acknowledgement of your support, this book is dedicated to you.

# CONTENTS

# ABBREVIATIONS

| | |
|---|---|
| BMA | British Medical Association |
| BMH | Bureau of Military History |
| CCS | Casualty Clearing Station |
| CMWC | Central Medical War Committee |
| FA | Field Ambulance |
| IMS | Indian Medical Service |
| IMWC | Irish Medical War Committee |
| IRA | Irish Republican Army |
| KOSB | King's Own Scottish Borderers |
| LGBI | Local Government Board for Ireland |
| MC | Military Cross |
| MO | Medical Officer |
| MOP | Ministry of Pensions |
| NUI | National University of Ireland |
| POW | Prisoner of War |
| QAIMNS | Queen Alexandra's Imperial Military Nursing Service |
| QAIMNSR | Queen Alexandra's Imperial Military Nursing Service Reserve |
| QUB | Queen's University Belfast |
| RAMC | Royal Army Medical Corps |
| RCPI | Royal College of Physicians of Ireland |
| RCSI | Royal College of Surgeons in Ireland |
| RMO | Regimental Medical Officer |
| RN | Royal Navy |
| SJA | St John's Ambulance |
| TCD | Trinity College Dublin |

| TFNS | Territorial Force Nursing Service |
| UCC | University College Cork |
| UCD | University College Dublin |
| VAD | Voluntary Aid Detachment |

# LIST OF FIGURES

# LIST OF TABLES

CHAPTER 1

# Introduction

In Ireland, the period from 1912 to 1925 was one of significant social and political change. The First World War was one of several major events that occurred during these years that affected the country and those who lived and worked in it. Support for the British war effort in Ireland, as elsewhere, was conditional. Immediately prior to the outbreak of war, the relationship between Britain and Ireland was undergoing considerable alteration. In 1912, British Prime Minister Herbert Asquith introduced the Third Home Rule Bill, which provided for an Irish parliament based in Dublin that would have had the authority to deal with most national affairs. Unionists, especially those in Ulster, were opposed to a Dublin-based administration. Consequently, political tensions rose to the extent that the outbreak of violence in Ireland appeared a real prospect. Both unionists and nationalists established paramilitary groups, escalating tensions in Ireland. The onset of the First World War in 1914 brought about the suspension of Home Rule. On 18 September 1914, the Suspensory Act received royal assent, which postponed the introduction of Home Rule until the war had ended.[1]

While Home Rule was postponed, the outbreak of violence in Ireland was not averted. On 24 April 1916, the Easter Rising—an armed insurrection—began and lasted for six days. Then, separatist nationalists organised the Rising in an attempt to end British rule in Ireland. Members of the Irish Volunteers and the Irish Citizen Army seized several locations in Dublin, including the General Post Office, and

© The Author(s) 2019
D. Durnin, *The Irish Medical Profession and the First World War*,
Medicine and Biomedical Sciences in Modern History,
https://doi.org/10.1007/978-3-030-17959-5_1

proclaimed an Irish Republic. The British Army suppressed the Rising with their superior military numbers and the insurgents agreed to surrender on Saturday 29 April. In the months that followed, British authorities ordered the execution of sixteen of the leaders of the rebellion.[2] It was against this backdrop of political upheaval and the rebellion in Ireland that the British government sought to encourage Irish men and women to support the British war effort and enlist in the various branches of the British Army.

For much of the twentieth century, historians largely ignored Irish involvement in the First World War. In 1967, F. X. Martin argued that Ireland was suffering from a national amnesia regarding its role in the First World War.[3] Martin's declaration followed the commemorations of the fiftieth anniversary of the 1916 Easter Rising and was prompted by the reluctance among many to acknowledge the large numbers of Irish people who participated in the British Army to serve in the war. Since then, Paul Fussell, Nuala Johnson and others have argued that the political agitation and violent conflict that occurred in Ireland following the end of the war were primarily responsible for this neglect.[4]

However, Martin's declaration can no longer be applied to Irish historiography. Significant historical work detailing the impact of the First World War on Ireland and the role of Irish people in the conflict has emerged over the past number of years. For example, since Martin's assertion, several historians have considered the impact of the war on Irish politics. Paul Bew, Thomas Hennessy and John Horne have argued that worldwide conflict altered the course of Irish politics by delaying Home Rule.[5] David Fitzpatrick has completed comprehensive work that establishes how the war disrupted everyday life.[6] Other studies have examined the rates and patterns of enlistment of Irish men into the combat forces of the military.[7] Estimates of the number of Irish who enlisted in the British Army during the First World War have varied considerably but Patrick Callan and Fitzpatrick have produced carefully considered assessments, which suggest that approximately 210,000 Irish personnel joined up.[8]

Academic research into the social and cultural history of medicine in Ireland has also grown considerably but, for the most part, themes relating to war and Irish medical provision remain relatively untouched.[9] This is in contrast with the vast amount of historical research on the British case, where a number of works have specifically focused on medicine and the First World War.[10] One of the first notable studies emerged in

1964, when Brian Abel-Smith, in his seminal study of the development of British hospitals from 1800 to 1948, argued that the standards of hospital care for civilians seriously declined because of the conflict.[11] Abel-Smith's negative assessment on the effect of war on civilian healthcare was unusual. From the 1960s to the end of the 1980s, other studies of the relationship between the war and medicine stressed the positive influence of conflict on medical innovation and provision. Rosemary Stevens posited that the First World War 'stimulated the development of special skills and special interests, particularly in psychiatry, orthopaedics, and plastic and thoracic surgery'.[12] Jay Winter argued that the war years were 'a period of significant gains in civilian health, for the young and those in the industrial labour force'.[13] Roger Cooter, in a typically astute study, later disputed the thesis that war was good for the development of medicine. He reasoned that studies dominated by this argument adopted a causal framework and that the theatres of war and medicine must be studied as part of the societies and cultures in which they were situated, something which most historical works on medicine and the First World War had lacked.[14] Cooter rejected the basic argument that the First World War benefited medicine and encouraged medical innovations as 'overtly positivist, implicitly militarist and profoundly simplistic'.[15]

More recent studies on the First World War and medicine have largely focused specifically on the provision of healthcare to soldiers. Mark Harrison, in his ground-breaking study, explored the role of the British Army medical services in the First World War and detailed the development of the casualty clearing process in multiple theatres of war, including the Western Front, Mesopotamia, Gallipoli and East Africa.[16] Emily Mayhew analysed the journey of wartime casualties from the battlefields to domestic hospitals in Britain.[17] Ian Whitehead's research focused specifically on the enlistment of medical officers (MOs) into the Royal Army Medical Corps (RAMC), a specialist corps responsible for providing medical care to all British Army personnel, to serve in the war and found that large numbers of doctors throughout Britain enlisted into the corps from 1914 to 1918.[18] All of these works have significantly enhanced our understanding of the British Army's medical arrangements during the First World War.

During the First World War, Irish medical personnel—physicians, surgeons, general practitioners and nurses—served in the medical services of the British Army. Yet a comprehensive history of Irish medical involvement in the conflict and its subsequent impact on the civilian medical profession does not exist.[19] This book analyses the extent of Irish medical involvement in the First World War and charts Irish medical personnel's enlistment from 1914 to 1918. It focuses primarily on physicians, surgeons and general practitioners who were born in Ireland. A considerable number of Irish nurses participated in the war and several historians have already explored their role in the conflict. In separate studies, Caitriona Clear, Siobhan Horgan-Ryan and Yvonne McEwen examined Irish nurses' wartime participation. Clear suggested that approximately 4500 of them served abroad during the war.[20] This book will examine the several different nursing services involved in the war and detail the wartime roles of Irish nurses to establish Irish medical experience on the frontlines. Unfortunately, the nature of the source material did not allow for a study of Irish nurses' enlistment rates and this is therefore not discussed. However, this provides scope for future research.[21]

It is argued here that many Irish medical personnel left behind their medical practices, hospital appointments and government posts to participate in the war and that the participation of the medical community affected Ireland's domestic medical infrastructure, including hospitals and general practices. In addition, several hospitals located throughout Ireland admitted British Army soldiers for treatment. This study explores the impact of worldwide conflict on Irish medical establishments, with a focus on hospitals and poor law medical services. In doing so, this book is an attempt to provide the first study of the effect of the First World War on Irish hospitals and civilian medical infrastructure.

This book is divided into seven chapters and focuses on medical provision and the Irish experience of the First World War from 1912 to 1925. These dates have been chosen to ensure that the study provides appropriate context to the effects of war on Irish medical provision. Extending the study to 1925 facilitates an analysis of developments in the years immediately after the war. It provides a sufficient time-scale to consider the immediate implications of political change in Ireland on the medical careers of Irish doctors who participated in the war. The end of hostilities on the Western Front did not signal the end of conflict for interwar Europe as violent upheavals and civil wars remained a characteristic feature of the region.[22] Ireland was no exception and experienced considerable political turmoil in the years after the First World War. In December 1918, Sinn Féin, an Irish republican political party, won a comprehensive victory in the Irish general election, which entitled them to seventy-three seats in the Imperial Parliament in

Westminster, London. However, Sinn Féin refused to recognise the parliament at Westminster and instead established an independent breakaway government—Dáil Éireann—and declared Irish independence from Britain. Violence and hostility between the Irish Republican Army (IRA), a republican military organisation; the Royal Irish Constabulary, the armed police force of the British state in Ireland, and the British Army, subsequently intensified and thus began the Irish War of Independence (1919–1921).[23]

On 3 May 1921, the Government of Ireland Act came into operation and divided Ireland into two jurisdictions—Northern Ireland and Southern Ireland—and elections for both Irish parliaments were held three weeks later.[24] Later, in December 1921, the government of the United Kingdom and Irish representatives signed the Anglo-Irish Treaty ending the Irish War of Independence and British rule in most of Ireland; Northern Ireland remained within the United Kingdom. This resulted in the creation of the Irish Free State, a self-governing state with dominion status. The signing of the treaty caused conflict between two opposing groups of Irish separatists—those in favour of accepting dominion status and those who saw it as a betrayal of the Irish republican cause. Consequently, in June 1922, a civil war erupted between the pro- and anti-treaty forces (1922–1923). A ceasefire was eventually called in the summer of 1923 following the exhaustion of the Anti-Treaty IRA's offensive abilities.[25] Against this background of partition, violence, domestic conflict and anti-British sentiment in the Irish Free State, many Irish doctors who had enlisted in the British Army for the First World War returned to Ireland—north and south—and sought to establish careers. This book is not concerned with the effect of partition and domestic conflict on health systems and the structure of the Irish medical profession, but rather the impact of conflict in Ireland on the careers of Ireland's returning wartime doctors.

Chapter 2 provides the necessary contextual framework for the study as well as a statistical analysis of Irish medical participation in the war. Philip Orr has argued that it is hard to be exact about the number of Irishmen who served with the British Army during the First World War.[26] The same is true for Irish medical personnel. However, using a variety of sources, it is possible to argue that approximately 3000 Irish doctors—physicians, surgeons and general practitioners—served in the British Army and associated medical services during the conflict.[27] A database based on a sample of 1800 was compiled for this study.[28]

For the purposes of Chapter 2, the database is used to provide details regarding the enlistment rates and years of enlistment. Due to the nature of the source material, it is not possible to provide monthly enlistment rates for Irish medical personnel into the British Army medical services and thus returns are given on an annual basis. This still allows the study to identify trends in Irish medical enlistment in the First World War and outline any alterations to these patterns as the war progressed.

Chapter 3 is concerned with the social profile of Irish medical personnel who joined up and examines the motivations behind their enlistment. The database comprises of biographical details including age, marital status and religious affiliation. A statistical analysis of this information produces detail on the background and educational characteristics of Irish medical volunteers.[29] This information is used to provide insight into their motivations for joining up. Using RAMC administrative records, as well as diaries and letters, this chapter also explores the wartime roles and experiences of Irish medical personnel, including nurses, in the First World War. Irish medics occupied several roles along the Army's system of casualty evacuation. An investigation of their experiences of these positions allows the study to determine whether they adapted to the difficult conditions of war and to evaluate whether the British Army treated Irish doctors differently due their nationality. In his study of Australian medical involvement in the First World War, Michael Tyquin has argued that cohesion and morale among Australian medics suffered as a consequence of the Australian Army Medical Corps' ill-defined and subservient role to the British Army medical services in Egypt and the Mediterranean.[30] Chapter 3 will analyse whether Irish doctors had similar problems with their British counterparts, particularly in the aftermath of the 1916 Easter Rising.

While this book utilises various collections of material to analyse Irish medical officers' wartime experiences, it focuses especially on four Irish doctors—James Johnston Abraham (1876–1963), Stafford Adye-Curran (1880–1928), Richard Hingston (1887–1956) and J. P. Lynch (1881–1948)—who authored comprehensive memoirs, diaries and letters during the conflict that describe their experiences in the various roles of the casualty dispersal process. Abraham was a surgeon who had a practice in London before enlisting in the British Army medical services for the duration of war, where he served in France. Hingston was a Regimental Medical Officer in the Indian Medical Services and served in several locations, including Basra. Both Adye-Curran and Lynch were career army medics in the British Army and served in the First World War. These four men occupied different roles in the British Army's medical clearing process and thus, a study of the sources authored by them offers an insight into the motivations behind Irish medical personnel's decision to enlist in the British Army medical services and details the roles and experiences of Irish medics during their time on the battlefields.[31]

An understanding of Irish nurses' experiences has been assembled from surviving accounts of several nurses but there is a focus on two case studies—Catherine Black (1883–1949) and Marie Martin (1892–1975). Black was a trained nurse who served in France. Martin was a Voluntary Aid Detachment nurse who served in Malta. A study of both Black and Martin gives a glimpse into the wartime experiences of both professional and VAD nurses during war. Black recorded her wartime experiences in her memoir *King's nurse, beggar's nurse*, which was published in 1939.[32] Martin documented her time at war in a series of letters sent to her mother during the conflict.[33] After the war, Black was appointed as nurse to King George V and Martin went on to establish the Medical Missionaries of Mary.

Chapter 4 moves away from studying personnel and instead focuses on hospitals. As part of the casualty evacuation process, the British Army used hospitals in Britain and Ireland to treat sick and wounded soldiers. Using hospital minute books, annual reports and other miscellaneous records, this chapter examines the RAMC's implementation of the casualty evacuation system in Ireland and analyses its impact on Ireland's network of hospitals—military and civilian. Chapter 4 is divided into two distinct time periods; the first details the development of the casualty clearing process and the impact it had on the civilian hospital system from 1914 to 1916. Harrison has argued that the RAMC altered their casualty evacuation process in 1916 and more sick and wounded soldiers were treated near the frontlines from 1916 onwards.[34] The second section of Chapter 4 explores the impact of this change, and continuing warfare, on the hospitals from 1916 to 1918.

Chapter 5 is concerned with the post-war career development of Irish medical personnel who had participated in the war. The process of medical demobilisation is examined to uncover whether doctors returned to Ireland and continued their pre-war occupations. It also explores whether the concerns of poor law boards of guardians and the Local Government Board regarding civilian health, especially after the outbreak of the influenza epidemic, accelerated the return of doctors to Ireland.

In addition, this chapter analyses whether the partition of Ireland, the Irish War of Independence and the Civil War influenced the career prospects of those who served with the British Army.

Chapter 6 explores the impact of the First World War on Ireland's hospitals in the years following the signing of the Armistice, up to 1925. Prior to 1914, Ireland's civilian hospitals were in a dire financial position and many were near to closure until the outbreak of conflict postponed decisions regarding their future. This chapter, building on the content of Chapter 4, determines whether hospitals—military, specialist and civilian—benefited from their involvement in the British Army's wartime medical infrastructure.

## MEDICAL ORGANISATIONS IN THE FIRST WORLD WAR

Irish doctors had enlisted into the British Army medical services long before the beginning of the First World War and throughout periods of amity. During the French Revolutionary and Napoleonic Wars, the number of doctors enlisted in the British Army significantly increased to form a dedicated British Army medical department. From the inception of this department to the years immediately prior to the outbreak of the First World War, British military command treated army MOs with little respect. For most of the nineteenth century, the War Office was opposed to granting military rank to medical men within the forces fearing that it could give medical personnel legitimate claim to command on the battlefield.[35] Peter Lovegrove has argued that the pay structure of the army created and fostered a divide between regular officers and medical men with regular officers receiving a higher wage than their medical counterparts.[36] Due to these divisions, military authorities often ignored army MOs' pleas for greater medical provision for the armed forces. Armed conflicts throughout the latter half of the nineteenth century were characterised by little or no medical support for British combat units. During the Crimean War (1853–1856), British troops had insufficient supplies of drugs. In addition, due to the lack of medical personnel to provide treatment, diseases such as typhus, dysentery and cholera spread with ease among combatants. In the seven months that followed the army's arrival in the Crimea, thirty-six per cent of the 28,000 men died from disease.[37]

Medical disasters during the Crimean conflict were described in detail in the *Times*, and these reports captured the attention of the public.[38]

Parliamentary committees and commissions were established to enquire into the lack of appropriate sanitation regulations among the forces and various recommendations for the improvement of the British Army medical services were implemented, including an increase in pay for medical personnel and the establishment of a new army medical school.[39] However, tension remained between regular military and medical personnel within the army. Army MOs sought to rectify this situation by attempting to secure legitimate military rank. Harrison has argued that this stemmed from the wider push for recognition among the British medical profession that had begun in the mid-nineteenth century.[40] The passing of the Medical Registration Act in 1858 and the growing influence of the British Medical Association (BMA) and its publication, the *British Medical Journal*, played a significant role in this clamour for recognition.[41] The BMA published a number of articles in the *British Medical Journal* calling for military authorities to recognise the importance of military MOs and were crucial in 'fighting the battle [for recognition] in all times and seasons'.[42]

The lack of respect and support from their military peers, coupled with the treacherous working environment on the battlefields, discouraged many medical men from joining the army medical services. Some medical schools, including Trinity College, Dublin (TCD), actively discouraged their students from enlisting. In 1878, at a specially convened conference, professors from TCD's School of Physic identified their perceived problems with the army medical services. According to them, the insistence on compulsory retirement after ten years' service and the military MO's lack of authority made service in the British Army an unattractive prospect for the medical man.[43] Throughout the 1890s, the BMA used their growing influence to pressurise the War Office to grant military rank to army medical personnel. Their attempts intensified following the medical disasters that occurred during the Boer Wars (1880–1881; 1899–1902) where once again, the shortage of medical personnel and a lack of knowledge regarding sanitation procedures among the troops led to severe outbreaks of disease.[44] In 1898, a meeting took place between the BMA and Lord Lansdowne, the Secretary of State for War, to discuss the issues concerning army medical men. The meeting culminated in the passing of a royal warrant ordering the amalgamation of the Army Medical Department and Army Hospital Corps into one newly formed organisation, the RAMC. The warrant also granted military rank to army medical personnel.[45]

In 1901, the Royal Commission appointed to investigate the treatment of the sick and wounded in South Africa—members included Sir Robert Romer, former Lord Justice of Appeal and Daniel John Cunningham, Chair of Anatomy, TCD—recommended further changes to the structure and practices of the army medical services.[46] They suggested permanently enlarging staff numbers and making provision for further enlargement in the case of war. The Commission argued that the efforts of Boer War MOs were commendable but a lack of numbers hampered their work and that an increase in the size of the RAMC would help combat the difficulties perpetuated by personnel shortage.[47] Due to the commission's report, various initiatives were introduced which aimed to boost the professional reputation and size of the corps; the RAMC made improvements to the conditions and training of MOs enlisted in the organisation and secured a new premises to house trainees. In 1903, the RAMC launched its own medical journal, the *Journal of the Royal Army Medical Corps*. The corps also implemented a number of recommendations, albeit slowly, concerning treatment for soldiers on the frontlines and in casualty clearing stations.[48]

Alfred Keogh, a County Roscommon native who had been Director-General of the RAMC from 1905, was heavily involved in the early twentieth-century changes to the RAMC. Keogh was educated at Queen's College, Galway and graduated with an MD and MCh (Master of Surgery) in 1878. He moved to London and held appointments in several hospitals before entering the British Army as surgeon in 1880. He served in the South African War, where his achievements led to promotion to the role of Deputy Director General of the corps and eventually to the position of Director.[49] Keogh visited a significant number of British hospitals and encouraged staff to prepare to undertake temporary commissions in the event of war.[50] He retired from the service in 1910.

His successor, Sir William Launcellotte Gubbins, who was born in County Limerick and educated at TCD, continued Keogh's initiatives. Gubbins' distinguished record of service in Afghanistan, Egypt, Burma, South Africa and India led to a string of consecutive promotions in the British Army medical services. He served as Deputy-Director under Keogh and was well placed to take up the mantle of Director following Keogh's retirement.[51] Under Gubbins' stewardship, the corps increased its number of permanent members and built a sizeable reserve of medical personnel to call upon in the case of a national emergency. Gubbins oversaw the introduction of various sanitation initiatives within the

British Army, including the introduction of anti-typhoid inoculation for recruits.[52] This was encouraged by the losses accrued in South Africa due to the disease and the apparent effectiveness of inoculation during various campaigns in India.[53] Gubbins retired shortly before the start of the First World War in 1914 and was replaced by Arthur Sloggett. Gubbins' contribution, along with Keogh's legacy, ensured that the RAMC had significantly improved as an organisation immediately prior to the outbreak of war.

Besides the RAMC, several voluntary groups provided important assistance to the British Army during the First World War. Foremost among them was the British Red Cross Society, an organisation that had originated in the nineteenth century. Following the beginning of the Franco-Prussian War in 1870, Colonel Robert James Loyd-Lindsay, a recipient of the Victoria Cross in 1857, organised a meeting of influential figures, including Lord Granville, the British Government's Foreign Secretary, to form the British National Society for Aid to the Sick and Wounded in War.[54] The society gave aid to both armies during the war under the red-cross emblem. In 1905, the organisation re-formed as the British Red Cross Society and three years later, King Edward VII and Queen Alexandra, granted a royal charter to the society. As part of its reconstitution, the society established a new internal framework, which included local branches that extended throughout Britain. In 1909, a British Red Cross voluntary aid scheme began which resulted in the formation of voluntary aid detachments in every county in England. By 1911, the British Red Cross and the Order of St John, its wartime partner, had established and organised 659 detachments between them in Britain and approximately 20,000 personnel had volunteered.[55] A number of high-profile individuals, including Lady Helen Munro-Ferguson, daughter of the Marquess of Dufferin and Ava, advocated the extension of the British Red Cross to Ireland as part of the 1909 scheme.[56] Following the outbreak of the First World War, several high-profile individuals established branches of the British Red Cross in counties throughout Ireland, including Cork and Dublin. For instance, Lady Aberdeen, Ishbel Maria Gordon, wife of the Lord Lieutenant of Ireland, organised a public meeting in the lecture theatre of the Royal Dublin Society and the outcome of this meeting was the official formation of the Dublin City Branch of the British Red Cross.[57]

As well as relying on voluntary organisations to provide medical care, the British Army also depended on its nursing corps. British Military nursing services comprised of a number of different groups, including the Queen Alexandra's Imperial Military Nursing Service (QAIMNS), the Queen Alexandra's Imperial Military Nursing Service Reserve (QAIMNSR) and the Territorial Force Nursing Service (TFNS). Established in 1902, the QAIMNS had strict and well-defined entry criteria. Nurses who wished to enlist in the service required three years' medical and surgical training in a civilian hospital recognised by the QAIMNS's advisory board.[58] In addition, the QAIMNS required their nurses to have a certain social background. A recruitment flyer sent to Irish hospitals defined this as 'regards education, character and social status, she [the nurse] is a fit person to be admitted to the QAIMNS'.[59]

Formed in 1908, the QAIMNSR and TFNS did not focus as much on the character of the nurses but significant nursing experience was expected. Those who wished to enlist were required to have three years training in a recognised civilian hospital or infirmary.[60] At the beginning of the war, approximately 2300 military nurses were attached to the various nursing groups.[61] Voluntary Aid Detachments (VADs) who joined the British Red Cross Society and the Order of Saint John also provided nursing assistance throughout the war. Alison Fell and Christine Hallett have estimated that by the end of conflict over 70,000 women had served as VADs.[62] Focusing on Irish medical personnel involved in the nursing corps and the other various organisations detailed above, this study will thus explore the role and experiences of Irish medical personnel in the First World War.

## NOTES

1. For more on Irish Home Rule, see David Fitzpatrick, *Politics and Irish life 1913–21: Provincial experience of war and revolution* (Cork: Cork University Press, 1977); Alvin Jackson, *Ireland 1798–1998: Politics and war* (Oxford: Oxford University Press, 1999); Alvin Jackson, *Home Rule: An Irish history, 1800–2000* (New York: Oxford University Press, 2003); Gabriel Doherty (ed.), *The Home Rule crisis, 1912–1914* (Cork: Mercier Press, 2014).

2. Detailed studies on the Rising include Charles Townsend, *Easter 1916: The Irish Rebellion* (London: Penguin Books, 2006); Fearghal McGarry, *The Rising: Easter 1916* (Oxford: Oxford University Press, 2010); Padraig Yeates, *A city in wartime: Dublin 1914–18* (Dublin: Gill and Macmillan, 2011).

3. F.X. Martin, '1916—Myth, fact and mystery' in *Studia Hibernica*, no. 7 (1967), pp. 7–125.
4. For more on the history of Irish memory and commemoration of the First World War, see Paul Fussell, *The Great War and modern memory* (Oxford: Oxford University Press, 1975); Adrian Gregory, *The silence of memory, Armistice Day 1919–46* (Oxford: Berg, 1994); Jeffery, *Ireland and the Great War*; Nuala Johnson, *Ireland, the Great War and the geography of remembrance* (Cambridge: Cambridge University Press, 2003); Tom Burke, 'Rediscovery and reconciliation: The Royal Dublin Fusiliers Association' in John Horne and Edward Madigan (eds.) *Towards commemoration: Ireland in war and revolution 1912–23* (Dublin: Royal Irish Academy, 2013), pp. 98–104; Paul Clark, 'Two traditions and the places between', in Horne and Madigan (eds.) *Towards commemoration*, pp. 67–73; Heather Jones, 'Church of Ireland Great War remembrance in the south of Ireland: A personal reflection' in Horne and Madigan (eds.) *Towards commemoration*, pp. 74–82; Fintan O'Toole, 'Beyond amnesia and piety' in Horne and Madigan (eds.) *Towards commemoration*, pp. 154–161.
5. Paul Bew, *Ideology and the Irish question: Ulster unionism and Irish nationalism, 1912–16* (Oxford: Clarendon Press, 1994); Thomas Hennessey, *Dividing Ireland: World War I and partition* (London: Routledge, 1998); Paul Bew, 'The politics of war' in John Horne (ed.) *Our war: Ireland and the Great War* (Dublin: Royal Irish Academy, 2008), pp. 95–130; Fitzpatrick, *Politics and Irish life*; Jeffery, *Ireland and the Great War*; John Horne, 'Our war, our history' in Horne (ed.) *Our war*, pp. 1–34.
6. David Fitzpatrick, 'Home Front and everyday life' in John Horne (ed.) *Our war*; Fitzpatrick, *Politics and Irish life*.
7. Patrick Callan, 'Ambivalence towards the Saxon shilling: The attitudes of the Catholic church in Ireland towards enlistment during the First World War' in *Archivum Hibernicum*, no. 41 (1986), pp. 99–111; Patrick Callan, 'British recruitment in Ireland, 1914–18' in *Revue Internationale d'Histoire Militaire*, no. 63 (1985), pp. 41–50; Patrick Callan, 'Recruiting for the British army in Ireland during the First World War' in *Irish Sword*, no. 17 (1987), pp. 42–56; Tom Johnstone, *Orange, green and khaki: The story of Irish regiments in the Great War, 1914–18* (Dublin: Gill and Macmillan, 1992); Thomas Dooley, *Enlisting in the British Army during the First World War* (Liverpool: Liverpool University Press, 1995); David Fitzpatrick, 'The logic of collective sacrifice: Ireland and the British Army, 1914–18' in *Historical Journal*, no. 38 (1995), pp. 1017–1030; Timothy Bowman, 'The Irish recruiting campaign and anti-recruiting campaigns, 1914–18' in Bertrand Taithe and Tim Thornton (eds.),

*Propaganda: Political rhetoric and identity, 1300–2000* (Stroud: Sutton, 1999), pp. 223–238; Pauline Codd, 'Recruiting and responses to the war in Wexford' in David Fitzpatrick (ed.) *Ireland and the First World War* (Dublin: Lilliput Press, 1998), pp. 15–26.

8. Patrick Callan, 'Voluntary recruiting for the British Army in Ireland during the First World War' (PhD thesis, University College Dublin, 1984); David Fitzpatrick, *Ireland and the First World War* (Dublin: Lilliput Press, 1986); Keith Jeffery, *Ireland and the Great War* (Cambridge: Cambridge University Press, 2010).

9. For an overview of Irish medical historiography Elizabeth Malcolm and Greta Jones, 'Introduction' in Elizabeth Malcolm and Greta Jones (eds.), *Medicine, disease and the state in Ireland, 1650–1940* (Cork: Cork University Press, 1999), pp. 1–20; see Catherine Cox, 'A better known territory? Medical history and Ireland' in *Proceedings of the Royal Irish Academy, section c*, no. 113 (2013), pp. 341–362. Selected studies on Irish medical history include Catherine Cox and Maria Luddy (eds.), *Cultures of care in Irish medical history, 1750–1970* (Basingstoke: Palgrave Macmillan, 2010); Catherine Cox, *Negotiating insanity in the southeast of Ireland, 1820–1900* (Manchester: Manchester University Press, 2012); Catherine Cox and Hilary Marland (eds.) *Migration, health, and ethnicity in the modern world* (Basingstoke: Palgrave Macmillan, 2013); Mark Finnane, *Insanity and the insane in post-famine Ireland* (London: ACLS History E-Book Project, 1981); Caitriona Foley, *The last Irish plague: The great flu epidemic in Ireland, 1918–19* (Dublin: Irish Academic Press, 2011); Greta Jones, '*Captain of all these men of death': The history of tuberculosis in nineteenth and twentieth century Ireland* (Amsterdam: Rodopi, 2001); Laura Kelly, *Irish women in medicine, c.1880s–1920s: Origins, education and careers* (Manchester: Manchester University Press, 2012); Laura Kelly, *Irish medical education and student culture, c.1850–1950* (Liverpool: Liverpool University Press, 2017); Anne Mac Lellan and Alice Mauger (eds.), *Growing pains: Childhood illness in Ireland, 1750–1950* (Dublin: Irish Academic Press, 2013); Ian Miller, *Reforming food in post-famine Ireland: Medicine, science and improvement, 1845–1922* (Manchester: Manchester University Press, 2014); Pauline Prior (ed.), *Asylums, mental health care and the Irish, 1800–2010* (Dublin: Irish Academic Press, 2012). Studies which examine themes of warfare and medicine in an Irish context include Joanna Bourke, 'Effeminacy, ethnicity and the end of trauma: The sufferings of shell-shocked men in Great Britain and Ireland, 1914–39' in *Journal of Contemporary History* 35, no. 1 (2000), pp. 57–69; P.J. Casey, K.T. Cullen and J.P. Duignan, *Irish Doctors in the First World War* (Kildare: Irish Academic Press, 2015); David Durnin and Ian Miller (eds.), *Medicine, health and Irish*

*experiences of conflict, 1914–45* (Manchester: Manchester University Press, 2017); Eoin Kinsella, *Leopardstown Park Hospital, 1917–2017* (Dublin: Leopardstown Park Hospital, 2017); Trevor Parkhill, *The First World War Diaries of Emma Duffin: Belfast Voluntary Aid Detachment Nurse* (Dublin: Four Courts Press, 2014); Foley, *The last Irish plague.*

10. A selection of work includes Brian Abel-Smith, *The hospitals, 1800–1948* (London: Heinemann, 1964); Rosemary Stevens, *Medical practice in modern England: The impact of specialization and state medicine* (New Haven: Yale University Press, 1966); Roger Cooter, *Surgery and society in peace and war: Orthopaedics and the organization of modern medicine, 1880–1948* (London: Macmillan, 1993); Thomas P. Lowry, *The story soldiers wouldn't tell: Sex in the Civil War* (Mechanicsburg: Stackpole Books, 1994); Lesly A. Hall, "'War always brings it on': War, STDs, the military, and the civilian population in Britain, 1850–1950" in Roger Cooter, Mark Harrison and Steve Sturdy (eds.), *Medicine and modern warfare* (Atlanta: Clio Medica, 1999), pp. 205–224; Mark Harrison, 'Sex and the citizen soldier: Health, morals and discipline in the British Army during the Second World War' in Cooter, Harrison and Sturdy (eds.), *Medicine and modern warfare*, pp. 225–250; Erica Charters, 'Military medicine and the ethics of war' in *Canadian Bulletin for the History of Medicine* 27, no. 2 (2010), pp. 273–298. Works that focus specifically on the First World War include: Jay Winter, *The Great War and the British people* (London: Macmillan, 1985); Roger Cooter, 'Medicine and the goodness of war' in *Canadian Bulletin of Medical History*, no. 12 (1990), pp. 147–159; Joanna Bourke, *Dismembering the male: Men's bodies, Britain and the Great War* (London: Reaktion, 1999); Ian Whitehead, *Doctors in the Great War* (Barnsley: Pen and Sword, 1999); Mark Harrison, *The medical war: British military medicine in the First World War* (Oxford: Oxford University Press, 2010); Jessica Meyer, *Men of war: Masculinity and the First World War in Britain* (Basingstoke: Palgrave Macmillan, 2011); Emily Mayhew, *Wounded: From Battlefield to Blighty, 1914–1918* (Leicester: Thorpe, 2013).

11. Abel-Smith, *The hospitals*, p. 252.

12. Rosemary Stevens, *Medical practice in modern England: The impact of specialization and state medicine* (New Haven: Yale University Press, 1966), pp. 38–52.

13. Winter, *The Great War*, p. 153.

14. Cooter, 'Medicine and the goodness of war', p. 149.

15. Roger Cooter, *Surgery and society in peace and war: Orthopaedics and the organization of modern medicine, 1880–1948* (London: Macmillan, 1993), p. 105.

16. Harrison, *The medical war*, pp. 291–302.

17. Mayhew, *Wounded*, pp. 9–81.
18. Whitehead, *Doctors in the Great War*, pp. 32–90.
19. One notable work is Casey, Cullen and Duignan's, *Irish doctors in the First World War*, which is an expertly compiled biographical list of Irish doctors involved in the conflict. See P.J. Casey, K.T. Cullen and J.P. Duignan, *Irish doctors in the First World War* (Kildare: Irish Academic Press, 2015).
20. Siobhan Horgan-Ryan, 'Irish military nursing in the Great War' in Gerard Fealy (ed.) *Care to remember* (Cork: Mercier Press, 2005), pp. 89–101; Caitriona Clear, 'Fewer ladies, more women' in Horne (ed.) *Our war*, p. 162.
21. At the time of research, the structure of the source material for nursing in the First World War made it difficult to obtain any accurate statistics to reveal the extent of involvement of Irish nurses in the war. The QAIMNS records, held in the National Archives, Kew, are rich and contain service records of 15,000 women who had served with the corps during the First World War, including pensions claimed. However, these records were not sorted by the nurse's nationality and it was not possible to complete a thorough survey of them for this study. Thus, there is plenty of scope for future research here.
22. Robert Gerwarth, 'The continuum of violence' in Jay Winter (ed.), *The Cambridge history of the First World War: The state* (3 vols, Cambridge: Cambridge University Press, 2014), ii, 639.
23. Peter Hart, *The IRA and its enemies: Violence and community in Cork, 1916–23* (Oxford: Oxford University Press, 1998).
24. Michael Laffan, *The partition of Ireland, 1911–1925* (Dundalk: Dundalgan Press, 1983).
25. Hart, *The IRA and its enemies*, pp. 21–38.
26. Philip Orr, '200,000 volunteer soldiers' in Horne (ed.) *Our war*, p. 65.
27. Services include Royal Army Medical Corps, Indian Medical Service, Royal Navy. This figure has been compiled from several sources including newspapers, such as the *Irish Times, Irish Independent, Freeman's Journal*, as well as several others. Further sources included the Kirkpatrick Index (Royal College of Physicians of Ireland [Hereafter RCPI], TPCK/5/3); *War list and roll of honour of the National University of Ireland* (Dublin, 1919); *Ireland's memorial records, 1914–18: Being the names of Irishmen who fell in the Great European War* (Dublin, 1923); *British Medical Journal*, 1880–1945; William Drew, William Johnston and Alfred Peterkin, *Commissioned officers in the medical services of the British Army, 1660–1960* (London: Wellcome Historical Medical Library, 1968).
28. Database based on sources detailed in note 27. Hereafter referred to as Database of Irish medical officers in British forces who served in the First World War. Those chosen to be part of the sample database were

included due to the level of the strength of the source material, which detailed their social, educational and professional backgrounds. The database contains their names and the various service details including their occupation prior to the war, regiment, rank, awards and occupation immediately following war.

29. Sample size for figures and tables in Chapter 3 vary. Based on the strength of source material available, samples are randomly selected from the original database of 1800.

30. Michael Tyquin, *Little by little: A centenary history of the Royal Australian Army Medical Corps* (Canberra: Department of Defence Army History Unit, 2003), p. 130.

31. It is important to note here that the sources associated with these men and other members of the Irish medical profession who served have limitations. Martyn Lyons has argued that the realities of war were frequently absent from soldiers' correspondence because of censorship and that the purpose of correspondence was often not to reveal the truth so much as to disguise it; soldiers wrote letters they expected the censors to read. The letters of medical men also had to pass through the censorship process, which was introduced in the early weeks of the war. What they recorded also depended on whom they were writing to and Lyons has argued that letters were often intended to be opened in public and read aloud. Lyons' arguments can be applied to letters and postcards from Irish doctors. For more on the limitations of these sources, see Martyn Lyons, *The writing culture of ordinary people in Europe, c.1860–1920* (Cambridge: Cambridge University Press, 2013). Memoirs are also somewhat problematic sources. They were often published many years after the war and when a doctor's medical career had concluded. For instance, James Abraham wrote his memoir *A Surgeon's Journey* in 1957. Therefore, it was important to recognise that the time elapsed between the wartime years and writing may have influenced memory and motives. To overcome these limitations, where possible, information contained in letters and memoirs relevant to this study have been cross-checked against newspapers, medical journals and RAMC records.

32. Catherine Black, *King's nurse, beggar's nurse* (London: Hurst and Blackett, 1939).

33. Letters cited in Medical Missionaries of Mary (Hereafter MMM), *A Dream to follow: The story of Marie Helena Martin aged 23 to 33* (Dublin: MMM, 2010). Also available in MMM, Collection B/F/1.

34. Harrison, *The medical war*, p. 65.

35. Whitehead, *Doctors in the Great War*, p. 11.

36. Peter Lovegrove, *Not least in the crusade: A short history of the Royal Army Medical Corps* (Aldershot: Gale and Polden, 1951), p. 9.

37. Lovegrove, *Not least in the crusade*, p. 9.
38. Whitehead, *Doctors in the Great War*, p. 7.
39. Whitehead, *Doctors in the Great War*, p. 9.
40. Harrison, *The medical war*, p. 5.
41. Harrison, *The medical war*, p. 5.
42. Anon., 'The week' in *British Medical Journal*, s4-1, no. 95 (1858), p. 889.
43. Anon., 'Army medical department' in *British Medical Journal*, 904, no. 1 (1878), p. 615.
44. For more detail on the medical disasters of the Boer Wars, see Lovegrove, *Not least*; Philip Curtin, *Disease and empire: The health of European troops in the conquest of Africa* (Cambridge: Cambridge University Press, 1998); Peter Prime, *The history of the medical and hospital services of the Anglo-Boer War, 1899–1902* (Chester: Anglo-Boer War Philatelic Society, 1998); Harrison, *The medical war*, p. 6.
45. Harrison, *The medical war*, p. 5.
46. Harrison, *The medical war*, p. 7.
47. Anon., 'Summary of the Royal Commission on South African Hospitals' in *British Medical Journal*, 2091, no. 1 (1901), p. 236.
48. Harrison, *The medical war*, p. 7.
49. Anon., 'Sir Alfred Keogh' in *British Medical Journal*, 3944, no. 2 (1936), p. 317.
50. Harrison, *The medical war*, p. 8.
51. Anon., 'Sir William Launcelotte Gubbins' in *British Medical Journal*, 3371, no. 2 (1925), p. 274.
52. Whitehead, *Doctors in the Great War*, p. 21.
53. Lovegrove, *Not least*, p. 12.
54. A.K. Loyd, *An outline of the history of the British Red Cross Society from its foundation in 1870 to the outbreak of the war in 1914* (London: British Red Cross Society, 1917).
55. Susan Cohen, *Medical services in the First World War* (London: Bloomsbury Publishing, 2014), p. 5.
56. *Irish Independent*, 18 August 1910.
57. *Irish Times*, 10 November 1914; *The Red Cross in Ireland: An account of the Red Cross Work of the St. John Ambulance Brigade and the British Red Cross Society in the provinces of Leinster, Munster and Connaught from August 1st, 1914 to November, 1918* (Dublin, 1919), p. 159; Ann Matthews, 'Cumann na mBan and the Red Cross, 1914–16' in R.V. Comerford and Jennifer Kelly (eds.), *Associational culture in Ireland and the wider world* (Dublin: Irish Academic Press, 2010), p. 182. Dame Ishbel Maria Gordon, marchioness of Aberdeen and Temair, philanthropist was married to John Campbell Gordon, 7th earl of Aberdeen.

In 1905 Aberdeen was reappointed as Lord Lieutenant by the new liberal government and Ishbel undertook much charitable work. Lady Aberdeen was associated with public health campaigns, including the anti-tuberculosis campaign led by the Women's National Health Association (WNHA). She continued her relationship with philanthropic healthcare movements in the early part of the First World War, most notably through her relationship with the Red Cross.

58. Horgan-Ryan, 'Irish military nursing in the Great War', p. 89.
59. Horgan-Ryan, 'Irish military nursing in the Great War', p. 89.
60. Horgan-Ryan, 'Irish military nursing in the Great War', p. 89.
61. Alison S. Fell and Christine E. Hallett, 'Introduction' in Alison S. Fell and Christine E. Hallett (eds.), *First World War nursing: New perspectives* (London: Taylor & Francis, 2013), p. 1.
62. Fell and Hallett, *First World War nursing*, p. 2.

# CHAPTER 2

# Recruitment and Irish Medical Personnel, 1914–1918

'I am afraid I was vain enough to think that that my action in going to France would meet with approval from the [Rotunda Hospital] Board rather than their calls for my resignation, particularly in view of the great slackness with regard to war which exists in Ireland'.[1]

On 1 August 1914, Arthur Sloggett, the newly appointed Director General of the RAMC, requested that the Dean and Registrar of the Royal College of Physicians of Ireland 'inform him confidentially as to the probable number of junior medical graduates in touch with the Royal College who would be likely to accept temporary service in the army for attachment to the RAMC in the event of a national emergency'.[2] Sloggett's request followed a similar appeal from the Director General of the Royal Navy Medical Department, who called on the college to 'recommend young qualified practitioners to volunteer for service in the Royal Navy should it be necessary to mobilise the fleet'.[3] Sloggett received a swift response stating that while the College acknowledged the appeal, they were 'unable to furnish any names of candidates at the present time'.[4] This response, coupled with the criticism from Henry Jellett, Master of the Rotunda Hospital in Dublin, quoted at the opening of this chapter, implies that members of the Irish medical profession were slow to enlist into the British Army medical services following the outbreak of the First World War.[5]

© The Author(s) 2019

D. Durnin, *The Irish Medical Profession and the First World War*,
Medicine and Biomedical Sciences in Modern History,
https://doi.org/10.1007/978-3-030-17959-5_2

However, to date, there has yet to be a study that examines the enlistment trends among the Irish medical profession. Winter and Whitehead have analysed the enlistment of doctors in England, Scotland and Wales into the British Army, and have suggested that more than half of the British medical profession enlisted by 1918.[6] They have also scrutinised the work of the Central Medical War Committee, the primary committee in Britain for recruiting medical personnel into the British Army medical services, and have argued that the committee played a crucial role in the recruitment of doctors into the army.[7] This chapter will examine the enlistment of Irish doctors into the British Army medical services in the First World War. Its main concern is to analyse the process of medical recruitment and uncover how it was managed in Ireland. It will therefore explore the impact of the establishment of the Irish Medical War Committee on the recruitment of Irish doctors.

## Early Recruitment Campaigns

On 4 August 1914, when Britain formally declared war, the RAMC immediately deployed a significant contingent of medical personnel, including 900 MOs, 10,000 other ranked members of the RAMC and 600 military nurses, to accompany the British Expeditionary Force. It was the largest medical contingent of any force that had left Britain.[8] Despite this, it soon became apparent that the RAMC was significantly understaffed for the demands of war. Early engagements, such as the Battle of Mons in August 1914, highlighted the inadequacies of the RAMC and the pressure on the corps. Eugene Ryan, a County Cork doctor who was Douglas Haig's personal medical officer in the early stages of the war, maintained that the medical staff were under severe pressure during the retreat from Mons, noting that he 'went to the [local] hospital which I found full of wounded … and the Germans were on our heels'.[9] To alleviate the RAMC's heavy workload and the shortage of doctors, the War Office sought to recruit more civilian medical personnel into the corps.[10] Ireland, with its overstocked medical profession, provided the War Office with a considerable pool of potential recruits.

On 6 August 1914, Trinity College Dublin, the Royal College of Surgeons in Ireland and the Apothecaries' Hall of Ireland launched the first medical recruitment campaign of the war in Ireland. They publicly requested recently qualified medical practitioners, who were not in permanent employment, to send their details—names and educational qualifications—to the registrars of these institutions. The registrars forwarded the applicants' details to the War Office, who then offered commissions to the doctors.[11] In contrast to the claims made by Henry Jellett in November 1914, an article in the *British Medical Journal* asserted that the Irish response to the early recruitment campaign was 'large and immediate' as sixty doctors applied for commissions within a day of the pleas appearing in the press.[12]

These claims of a quick and considerable response are borne out in the sample of Irish medical recruits examined.[13] Twenty per cent of doctors who participated in the conflict enlisted and began serving with the corps between the beginning of the war and 31 December 1914 (Fig. 2.1). This was the most active period of enlistment among Irish doctors during the conflict.[14] The initial support for the war demonstrated by Irish doctors was comparable to that of Irishmen joining the combat forces of the British Army. Patrick Callan has shown that the first six months of the war were the peak period for Irish enlistments into the non-medical forces of the British Army.[15]

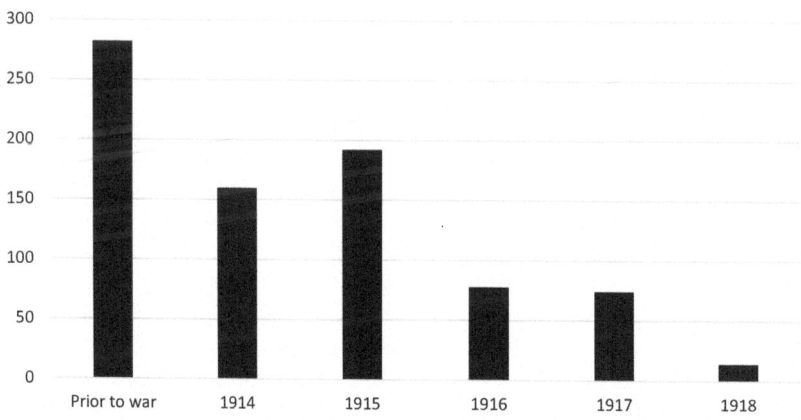

**Fig. 2.1**  Enlistment rates of Irish doctors who served in the First World War (*Source* Database of Irish medical officers in British forces who served in the First World War—based on sample of 800 doctors [Sample size based on those in the Database of Irish medical officers in British forces who served in the First World War with the most accurate enlistment information])

From early 1915, as the need for additional manpower in the British Army increased, the War Office introduced a number of new initiatives to raise Irish recruitment levels including the appointment of Lord Wimborne, veteran of the Second Boer War, as specialised Director of Recruiting for Ireland.[16] On the outbreak of war, Wimborne had joined the staff of Lieutenant General Sir Bryan Mahon who was commanding a division at the Curragh Barracks in County Kildare. Shortly afterwards, on 16 February 1915, Wimborne was appointed Lord Lieutenant of Ireland, a position he held until 1918.[17] By 1915, the position of Lord Lieutenant to Ireland had become a largely ceremonial role.[18] However, Guest sought to actively contribute to the war and as Director of Recruiting for Ireland, he oversaw the implementation of various new procedures to develop relationships and coordination between existing central and local recruitment committees. A Department of Recruiting was organised with several provincial directors of recruiting appointed and local recruitment committees formed or reorganised.[19] Ireland was divided into six administrative regions—Connaught, Donegal, East, North, Southeast and Southwest—and local county councillors were made responsible for recruitment campaigns in their regional division. The recruitment of medical personnel largely fell outside Guest's remit and was primarily left to the medical profession, particularly the Irish branch of the British Medical Association (BMA), to organise among themselves.

From the early stages of war, the BMA had been central to the medical recruitment process in Britain. Medical recruitment in Britain was largely characterised by a system of self-government and BMA initiatives remained relatively untouched by the War Office and the Ministry of National Service.[20] Instead, the BMA orchestrated recruitment and used its influence and official publications to encourage their members to enlist in the RAMC. In early 1915, the BMA established a Medical Emergency Committee based on similar pioneering committees formed by medical professionals in Scotland.[21] The Medical Emergency Committee met sporadically and discussed various issues relating to the British medical profession's role in the war, including recruitment and the impact of the conflict on domestic medical services. The War Office hierarchy and the medical profession were keen to ensure that the enlistment of doctors into the British Army medical services did not jeopardise civilian medical provision. Consequently, as the need for medical personnel in the British Army increased, the BMA established a dedicated committee to deal with these issues.

On 31 July 1915, the BMA formed the Central Medical War Committee, which sought to encourage members of the medical profession in England, Wales and Ireland to enlist in the RAMC.[22] Committee members included the heads of medical educational institutions and licencing bodies. Dr. Thomas Hennessy, fellow of the Royal College of Surgeons in Ireland, represented the Irish medical profession on the committee.[23] Hennessy practised as a dispensary doctor for over twenty years in Clogheen, a rural village in County Tipperary, before becoming the Irish Medical Secretary of the BMA in 1914.[24] While Hennessy's position on the Central Medical War Committee ensured that Irish medical personnel had representation on the board, his involvement with the committee was minimal. It was not feasible for Hennessy to travel to England to attend the meetings regularly and his attendance was primarily limited to annual general meetings.[25] Instead, Hennessy was heavily involved on another wartime committee—the Irish Medical War Committee.

The Central Medical War Committee had encouraged a steady stream of medical enlistments throughout 1915 and to achieve maximum results and efficiency regarding recruitment, it established subsidiary groups to cover various regions throughout the United Kingdom. The Irish Medical War Committee was established under this initiative. Ephraim Cosgrave, President of the Royal College of Physicians of Ireland, chaired the committee. Other prominent members included: D. J. Coffey, President, University College Dublin; A. F. Dixon, Dean of Faculty of Physic, Trinity College Dublin; F. Conway Dwyer, President, Royal College of Surgeons in Ireland; Joseph O'Carroll, Vice-President, Royal College of Physicians of Ireland and William Taylor, Vice-President, Royal College of Surgeons in Ireland.[26] Thomas Hennessy and Maurice Hayes, a graduate of the Catholic University Medical School, acted as secretaries. The Irish Committee was largely self-governing but shared common objectives with the Central Medical War Committee, most notably ensuring that a significant number of medical personnel enlisted with the RAMC for war service.

To achieve this aim, the Irish Medical War Committee took responsibility for both the wartime enrolment scheme for doctors and medical recruitment campaigns in Ireland. Medical professionals, who declared themselves available for war service, enrolled with the Irish Medical War Committee. The committee added the details of volunteers to a register and assessed whether candidates were suitable for enlistment into the

RAMC and then informed the candidate whether they were approved for active service.[27] The purpose of the enrolment scheme was to ensure that suitable candidates joined the British Army medical services and the enlistment of medical personnel did not undermine the quality of civilian medical services.

To encourage enlistment, the Irish Medical War Committee issued regular appeals to doctors. On 8 November 1915, at one of the first meetings of the Irish Medical War Committee, the group sent a circular letter to every member of the medical profession up to the age of forty-five—the age limit for war service in the medical corps—urging them to volunteer for the RAMC. The committee identified workhouse and dispensary medical officers as a potential pool of recruits.[28] These medical officers were employed as part of the Irish poor law system, under the 1851 Medical Charities Act.[29] Poor law appointments were highly valued and provided financial security to the holder.[30] Fearing that their jobs would not be available on their return, poor law medical officers were thus understandably reluctant to vacate their posts to participate in war.

To entice medical officers to leave their position temporarily to participate in the war, it was important that the Irish Medical War Committee could offer them a level of job protection while they were abroad. To achieve this, the committee encouraged those enlisting to nominate their own replacements—*locum tenentes*—to cover for them while they were serving abroad. This was not a new practice in Ireland; for decades, a system of nomination had allowed Irish medical officers to protect their posts.[31] The committee also sought the cooperation of national and local bodies responsible for the employment of medical officers—the Local Government Board for Ireland (LGBI) and poor law boards of guardians—in their efforts to safeguard the jobs of doctors joining the RAMC.[32] Established in 1872, the LGBI administered the Irish poor law and the boards of guardians.[33] With regard to the appointment of medical officers, while guardians hired doctors to the various poor law dispensary district posts, the LGBI sanctioned the appointments. On 20 November 1915, the Irish Medical War Committee requested the assistance of the guardians and LGBI:

> In view of the urgent need which exists for doctors to serve in the RAMC, the Irish Medical War Committee strongly urges Boards of Guardians and other corporations to facilitate their medical officers to the fullest extent of

volunteering their services. In furtherance of this object, the committee are of the opinion that public bodies should accept the substitutes nominated by their medical officers, provided that the interests of the sick poor are safeguarded to the satisfaction of the Local Government Board.[34]

The LGBI supported the Irish Medical War Committee's aims and on 26 November 1915, issued a letter to the clerk of each union in Ireland informing guardians not to make new and permanent medical appointments during the war as it was 'inequitable to the doctors who, out of the motives of patriotism and humanity, have placed their services for the time being at the disposal of the Government'.[35]

The Irish Medical War Committee also encouraged medical personnel that were not employed in state posts to enlist. The committee specifically targeted educational institutions to advise newly qualified doctors to join the RAMC. With prominent figures from Irish medical education on the committee, this proved a logical and relatively uncomplicated process. Members of staff at educational institutions, including the Royal College of Physicians of Ireland, Royal College of Surgeons in Ireland and Queen's University, Belfast, urged medical students to enrol in the RAMC immediately after graduation. At the conclusion of a spring graduation ceremony at Queen's University, Belfast, Dr. Leslie, President of the Ulster Medical Society, made a long address in which he strongly appealed to the newly qualified students to join the RAMC declaring that 'never was a bigger urgency for doctors of military age to join the RAMC'.[36] The recruitment figures demonstrate that newly qualified Irish medical personnel eagerly enlisted into the RAMC. For instance, in the RCSI's 1915 graduating class, eighty-seven per cent of the graduates enlisted in the RAMC.[37] Similar patterns were evident in medical schools throughout Ireland.

There were three primary reasons for the success of this initiative. Firstly, the RAMC was a readily available career option for newly qualified students seeking employment. Secondly, aside from a difficult period in the 1870s, the enlistment of newly qualified medical students into the RAMC and other associated bodies was a long-standing tradition that continued during wartime. Finally, following the outbreak of war, nearly all the licencing bodies in Ireland held supplemental examinations so that students who wished to enlist could sit their final exams as quickly as possible.[38] According to Charles Benson, assistant surgeon at Sir Patrick Dun's Hospital in Dublin, 'this undoubtedly had the effect of speeding up the senior students who on receiving their qualifications were able to offer themselves for commissions in the naval and army medical services'.[39]

## 1916 AND THE DECLINE IN ENLISTMENT

By 1916, the enlistment rates of Irish doctors began to slow (Fig. 2.1). As Keith Jeffery has argued, there is no 'monocausal explanation' to account for the alterations in the pattern of Irish enlistment rates in the British Army during the First World War.[40] Instead, there are a number of plausible explanations for peaks and troughs and the same is true for the enlistment patterns of Irish doctors. In April 1916, members of the Irish Volunteers and Irish Citizen Army embarked upon an armed insurrection—the Easter Rising—against British rule in Ireland. As enlistment rates of Irish men into the British Army began to decline around this time, several historians have analysed the effects of the Rising on recruitment. Patrick Callan has suggested that the impact of the Rising on recruitment was minimal and that enlistment rates into the combat forces of the British Army were already on the decline prior to the Rebellion.[41] David Fitzpatrick has argued that there was a resurgence in recruitment figures during the months following the Rising due to an increase in loyalism towards Britain among sections of the Irish population.[42] The subsequent rise in Irish enlistment into the combat forces in 1918 certainly casts doubt on any detrimental link between the Rising and Irish recruitment rates.[43]

As Fig. 2.1 demonstrates, a later rise in medical recruitment rates never transpired. Instead, Irish medical enlistment rates in the British Army declined in 1916, a downward trend that continued for the duration of the war. There is evidence that the Rising encouraged a small number of medical students to quit their medical studies to enlist into the British Army as regular combatants. Michael Taaffe, a TCD medical student, recalled in his memoirs that the outbreak of the Rising in Dublin encouraged him to join the British Army:

> When my third term at Trinity had come to an end, I had walked into a dingy office not far from Westland Row to enlist … I hadn't it was true, awakened one morning with my mind made up, but ever since the first day of the rebellion, when I had seen the young officer of the Leinster Regiment sheathe his sword and walk unhurriedly through the gate of Trinity, I had known what I must do.[44]

Taaffe dropped out of his medical course and enlisted in an artillery regiment. He claimed he was not alone:

> On me and my kind the Rebellion had two immediate effects. It determined the future for a lot of us and turned us, for the time being, into anarchists of a minor order. In bringing war to our doorstep it had also brought the war in France closer and most of the men in my year, whether they were conscious of it or not, had made up their minds to join one of the Services as soon as they had got credit for the term. A few, unable to wait longer, slipped away quietly in the weeks immediately following the end of the Rebellion, and among those of us who remained, our thoughts all in the exciting future, discipline grew slack.[45]

It is therefore possible that the Irish Rebellion prompted a decline in Irish medical recruits as medical students who were prospective RAMC recruits instead dropped their studies in favour of an immediate enlistment into the combat regiments of the British Army. It is, however, more likely that several other factors were responsible for the decline in medical enlistments.

After the early battles of the war, men enlisting in the regular regiments of the army returned home for routine rest or for medical treatment and shared stories of their experiences with their contemporaries.[46] Their accounts detailed the harsh realities of war and they may have discouraged others from enlisting. In addition, many doctors on war service complained of having heavy administrative workloads, which often prevented them from treating the sick and wounded.[47] Other doctors protested that the RAMC assigned them to locations where medical expertise was not required. In 1915 the RAMC had assigned Dr. Stafford Adye-Curran, who was educated at the Catholic University, Dublin, and joined the RAMC in 1901 after a stint as a civil surgeon in South Africa, to Rouen, France.[48] He later complained that there was 'nothing to be done in the way of work' during his time there.[49]

General practitioners also became reluctant to enlist as the practices of those who had already enlisted started to fail. In the early stages of war, doctors who remained in Ireland had pledged to protect the private practices of those who enlisted. In 1915, for instance, Dr. Peter McKenna in County Monaghan called on his fellow medical practitioners in the county to band themselves together to facilitate those who wished to enlist and 'protect and preserve the practice and appointments of any such member'.[50] Like poor law medical officers, general practitioners also arranged for locums to undertake their duties. Nevertheless, as the war progressed those who had agreed to protect fellow doctor's practices enlisted themselves and it became increasingly difficult for doctors to secure a colleague to act as locum for the duration of the conflict. In November 1915, Charles Benson signalled growing problems with the locum system and insisted that 'in civil practice, a *locum tenen* was almost unobtainable'.[51] By 1916, the *Irish Times* reported that general practitioners who had enlisted had 'sacrificed their practices ... to the national need'.[52]

Irish doctors were also reluctant to enlist after the end of the initial waves of enthusiasm because of increased employment opportunities in Ireland and Britain. War was 'good for business' for Ireland's doctors, at least for the period 1914–1918. Those who vacated their jobs to join the RAMC in the early months of the war freed up opportunities for other medical personnel in Ireland. In 1914, for example, Hugh Grant, a newly qualified doctor who graduated with a L. M. from the Coombe Hospital, part of the Catholic University in Dublin, was appointed by the Newry Board of Guardians in County Down as MO for a Newry rural district after the incumbent, Dr. H. W. Smartt, enlisted in the RAMC. Grant retained the position until Smartt returned, gaining medical experience and utilising the opportunity to establish his own private practice in Newry.[53] Women doctors especially benefited from the departure of medical men for war. Winter has posited that in Britain the number of women doctors in the medical profession grew during the First World War as opportunities, previously unavailable to them, opened up.[54] A similar trend emerged in Ireland.[55] In 1916, Dr. Charles Benson of Sir Patrick Dun's Hospital in Dublin, claimed that

> The war has given women an opportunity of proving their mettle, and that they have taken it with earnest enthusiasm is common knowledge ... war has had the effect of levelling many prejudices, and not least among them is that against the women members of our profession, many of whom have been successful candidates for appointments hitherto not open to them.[56]

This rush to fill vacant posts discouraged enlistment as it caused considerable concern for doctors, who feared that should they enlist in the British Army, their jobs or practice would no longer be available on return. Such concern was evident among English doctors who had already enlisted in the RAMC and were concerned about the security of their jobs partly because of the influx of Irish doctors into the region. Along with doctors from other countries including India, China, Portugal and Egypt, Irish doctors travelled to occupy the vacant posts that became available throughout Britain.[57] An anonymous English physician, who was a captain in the RAMC, complained in a letter to the *British Medical Journal* that the number of British medical professionals enlisting in the war effort left 'it open to young Irish practitioners to profit and set up practice in the homes of the English, Scottish and Welsh absentees, to their obvious hurt'.[58]

Doctors who remained in Ireland during the first year of war often emphasised that they simply could not enlist due to the sheer volume of medical work in their home districts. By late 1915, doctors in various parts of Britain, including Coventry and Nottingham, had expressed concern that their jobs had become stressful due to an increase in their workload as a consequence of colleagues enlisting in the RAMC.[59] Doctors who remained in Ireland voiced similar worries. In April 1915, Dr. John Mills, assistant resident medical superintendent to the Ballinasloe Asylum, requested the asylum governors permit him to volunteer for the RAMC. While the governors permitted Mills to leave, his colleagues expressed concerns about the effect of his enlistment on the workings of the asylum. At a specially convened meeting of the asylum governors and medical staff, Dr. James Kirwan, resident medical superintendent, expressed concerns about Mill's potential departure: 'all the work will have to fall on Dr. [Ada] English and myself'.[60] The chairman of the board of governors agreed with Kirwan and argued that 'we must keep a certain number of doctors in the country'.[61] Kirwan further contended that 'we all feel the call as well as Dr. Mills. All the glory is not with the man who goes out, as the man who stays at home can do as much good work as the next'.[62]

## CONSCRIPTION, REGULATION AND DISSENSION

As enlistment rates into both the combat and medical forces of the British Army began to slow, the War Office's need for manpower increased and legislation reflected this demand. In January 1916, the British government passed a new Military Service Act which provided for the conscription of single men aged from eighteen to forty-one years, while a further Act passed in May conscripted married men. There was strong opposition to conscription in Ireland. On 8 June 1915, the

Irish Parliamentary Party—the official parliamentary party for Irish nationalist members of parliament elected to the House of Commons in Westminster—had declared that they were opposed to compulsory military service because 'it is unnecessary, and because any attempt to enforce it would break up the unity of the people of these islands'.[63] Fears that conscription would disrupt the unity between Ireland and Britain were well founded. By 1916, anti-British sentiment, encouraged by fears regarding conscription, was growing in Ireland and it threatened to disrupt Irish support for the war and consequently reduce recruitment rates. For example, the north Meath executive of the United Irish League, a nationalist political party, resolved to oppose conscription and argued that it 'was the duty of the Irish members [enlisted in the Army] to come back and help Ireland to get Home Rule'.[64] Due to the political opposition to the act, most notably from the Irish Parliamentary Party, the British government did not extend conscription to Ireland.[65]

As far as Ireland's medical personnel were concerned, debates regarding their conscription ultimately mattered little after discussions between the War Office and the Central Medical War Committee ensured that both Irish and British medical personnel were exempt from conscription. It was decided that it was best for the medical war committees to continue to manage medical recruitment. The *Irish Times*, an ardent supporter of conscription in Ireland, encouraged Irish doctors to insist on a reversal of this decision and seek conscription for their own profession. According to an article that appeared in the newspaper in December 1916, conscription had the potential to end the problem of doctors, who remained in Ireland, setting up private practices in the localities of those who had departed for war. The anonymous author of the article argued that

> so far as Irish doctors are concerned a decision in favour of compulsion – at least for doctors of military age – by our own Colleges of Physicians and Surgeons would have much weight. Many of us know of cases where the practices of young Irish doctors who have joined the Army have fallen, in whole or part, into the hands of equally young men who preferred to stay at home.[66]

Instead of pressing for the introduction of conscription, both the Irish Medical War Committee and the Central Medical War Committee decided to persevere with the enrolment scheme and launched new initiatives to encourage medics' enrolment.

Firstly, following the passing of the Military Act that introduced conscription, the Army Council issued an official order, published in the *British Medical Journal*, which stated that 'no medical practitioner willing to accept, if offered, a commission in the RAMC should be accepted as an ordinary combatant'.[67] Doctors were a valuable commodity to the domestic medical infrastructure and the War Office agreed that it would be unwise to allow medical practitioners to enlist as ordinary combatants in the army. Secondly, in March 1916, the Local Government Board in England and Wales informed boards of guardians that it was necessary to make 'provisional arrangements for enabling every medical man of suitable age (45 and under) who could be spared from civil employment without serious injury to the civil population, to place himself at the disposal of the authorities and to be prepared, if required, to take a commission in the Army or Navy in the near future'.[68] On request from the Central Medical War Committee, the Local Government Board instructed boards of guardians to classify their medical officers under three headings—those who could be spared at once; those who might be spared later; and those who cannot be spared—and inform the committee of their findings.[69] By using these lists, the Central Medical War Committee could identify suitable potential recruits and encourage their enrolment without wholly damaging local health services.

In Ireland, the LGBI requested that guardians refrain from appointing doctors of military age and, crucially, announced that they [the LGBI] would refuse to sanction payment to any doctor appointed, even temporarily, who was of military age. There was notable discern among sections of the Irish medical profession to this ruling as it limited doctors' employment options, and essentially stopped doctors of military age, albeit with a few exceptions, from securing employment in the poor law medical services. The *Medical Press* accused the LGBI of 'forcing Irish doctors into the army' and that 'distinctions were being drawn between Irish medical men and the rest of their fellow citizens'.[70] Boards of guardians throughout Ireland were also concerned about the decision as it limited their choice of candidates for medical posts. Offering what it thought was a practical solution, the LGBI advised guardians to assign posts to local doctors holding another permanent appointment or to divide the duties between two or more medical officers. According to the LGBI, guardians could only appoint a new medical officer as a last resort and in that case, they were to be over military age.[71]

The LGBI's ruling intensified the fractious relationship between it and several boards of guardians, who had already begun to demonstrate a lack of support for the war effort which proved detrimental to Ireland's medical enlistment rates. In 1916, several poor law boards, including the Kenmare Board of Guardians in County Kerry and the Carrickmacross Board of Guardians in County Monaghan, cancelled or refused to allow the appointments of the temporary medical officers who had been nominated by those enlisting to serve as locums.[72] It is unclear why the guardians chose to cancel appointments; the nominated locums may have been unsatisfactory. Alternatively, it is likely that the decision was characteristic of the guardians' wider revolt against the LGBI. Most boards of guardians who openly defied the LGBI's efforts to encourage doctors to enlist into the British Army were largely composed of nationalist representatives who were hostile to LGBI interference in their decisions.

By 1916, Ireland's boards of guardians had become increasingly nationalist. Until the 1870s, a landowning class who were supportive of the Irish union with Britain had controlled Ireland's boards of guardians. Following the introduction of the various land acts in Ireland, however, tenants, many of whom supported Irish self-rule, acted collectively to exert their influence over local politics and steadily eroded the power of the landowning class.[73] The number of nationalists on poor law boards thus grew significantly. William Feingold has calculated that by 1886, tenant guardians made up approximately fifty per cent of office holders on poor law boards, compared to twelve per cent in 1877.[74] Consequently, Virginia Crossman has argued that there was a noticeable rise in nationalist sentiment among Ireland's poor law boards.[75]

Due to the rising number of nationalists on poor law boards, relations between guardians and the LGBI, a bastion of British rule in Ireland, became increasingly problematic and this was notable during the First World War. Crossman has posited that nationalists believed that the LGBI's insistence on a strict adherence to its rules was an attempt to hinder separatist campaigns.[76] The guardians' hostility towards the LGBI's stringent rules on wartime medical employment in the poor law services was thus likely an extension of wider opposition towards the LGBI's rules. In 1916, the Castlebar Board of Guardians, a predominantly nationalist board, complained about the LGBI's refusal to sanction the appointment of a new medical officer for the Balla dispensary district because he was of military age.[77] M. McGreevy, a member of the board, was angry that the LGBI refused to sanction the appointment given that the district had already lost another doctor who had enlisted into the RAMC; McGreevy asserted that 'we will not allow it. The people of Balla will not have it'.[78] Guardian A. Daly ultimately declared that 'the drones of the LGBI office can dictate to us alright, a safe distance from the war. I would like to see doctors going to the front, but … charity begins at home'.[79] Similar sentiments were evident at a meeting of the Killarney Board of Guardians in County Kerry. T. Brosnan, a member of the board, questioned whether the board 'were going to let the Local Government Board boss us?' and the chairman, Mr. O'Shea, agreed that the guardians should ignore the LGBI and stated that 'if the guardians supported these letters [from the LGBI], they were supporting conscription pure and simple'.[80] These disputes between the LGBI and guardians throughout Ireland continued but the LGBI was, for the most part, steadfast in its refusal to sanction any appointment of doctors of military age.

In 1917, the Lismore Board of Guardians, County Waterford, initiated legal proceedings against the LGBI over its refusal to sanction the appointment of a dispensary medical officer who was eligible for war service.[81] The Lismore Board, dominated by nationalist personnel, had a difficult relationship with the LGBI.[82] On 27 July 1917, the High Court heard the particulars of the case: Dr. Michael J. Kenny, Lismore dispensary medical officer, had taken a leave of absence due to illness. The Lismore Board of Guardians appointed Dr. John Dwyer, the medical officer of the adjoining Ballyduff dispensary, to cover for Dr. Kenny during his absence and the LGBI sanctioned Dwyer's appointment. Dr. Kenny, however, died from illness while on leave and the guardians advertised his job as a temporary position, available for the duration of the war. Three medical men who were of military age applied for the post. Dr. Thomas Cronin, a County Cork doctor, secured the position and the guardians made an application to the LGBI to sanction the appointment. On learning that Cronin was twenty-six years of age, the LGBI refused to authorise the appointment 'in view of the constant and increasing need for the services of medical men with His Majesty's Forces'.[83] The guardians argued that the LGBI had 'disregarded or subordinated to extraneous considerations, the provision of efficient medical relief for the sick poor of the dispensary district'.[84] The court ruled in favour of the LGBI, asking:

is it possible for us to pronounce a judicial condemnation of the action of the Local Government Board in providing for the economic "rationing" of the limited and decreasing supply of medical practitioners with a view to satisfy the pressing needs of the military service, without at the same time impeding or interfering with suitable and satisfactory arrangements for the medical relief of the sick poor? ... the Local Government Board would seem to have been dictated solely and simply by a regard for the admitted necessities of the country in the struggle for national existence through which it is passing.[85]

The Lismore case established a legal precedent, which provided the LGBI with a justification for their employment restrictions regarding doctors of military age and it was applied repeatedly in the years that followed. On 14 May 1917, the South Dublin Union Board of Guardians appointed Dr. E. B. Palmer as locum for a medical officer who was on temporary sick leave. The guardians requested the LGBI to sanction Palmer's payment but the LGBI refused because he was of military age and eligible for service with the RAMC. Thereupon, Palmer initiated legal proceedings against the LGBI. Despite winning the Lismore case, the LGBI decided to pay Palmer as 'the period of employment was short and the duties were discharged' but the LGBI reiterated that as a result of the judgement in the Lismore case, they would not be prepared to assent again to employment, 'even temporarily under the guardians of a doctor which is eligible for service with His Majesty's Forces, unless it can be conclusively proved that the guardians had no other option in order to safeguard the interests of the sick poor'.[86]

## MEDICAL RECRUITMENT IN THE FINAL YEARS OF WAR

By 1917, Ireland's contribution of medical personnel was largely in line with England, Scotland and Wales as approximately half of the medical profession had enlisted.[87] By the latter stages of war, Ireland could thus not afford to lose any more medical personnel to the military services without placing additional pressure on civilian medical provision, which was already suffering due to the shortage of doctors. Winter has posited that despite the absence of such a large percentage of doctors, there was no crisis in the provision of medical care in wartime Britain.[88] This was not the case in Ireland. Instead, the departure of such a considerable number of doctors undermined the provision of medical care in several regions, most notably in rural areas. Public representatives in various parts of rural Ireland reported that there was no doctor in their region. In November 1917, for example, the Cashel Board of Guardians in County Tipperary complained to the LGBI that the Fethard district— an area with a population of approximately 4000 people—was without a doctor because of the war.[89] Doctors from other districts had to travel to Fethard to provide medical care to those in the area but arrangements like this had been trialled in other counties and proved to be wholly unworkable due to the distance involved.[90]

As a consequence of the pressure on civilian medical infrastructure, the Irish Medical War Committee found it increasingly difficult to generate enough recruits to satisfy the demands of the RAMC, although they continued to issue appeals to doctors to enlist:

> it is realised that the existing needs of the population will put a strain on the remaining members of the profession, and will entail the cutting down of the medical services to the really essential. But it must be remembered that the needs of the wounded combatants have first claim on our services and the public must be prepared to do with less medical attendance just as they are having to restrict necessaries and deny themselves luxuries.[91]

The enlistment rates detailed in Fig. 2.1 show that these appeals had little impact.

In March 1918, the British Army suffered significant losses following the Spring Offensive on the Western Front; both men and ground were lost, with the Germans gaining approximately ninety-eight square miles of territory.[92] As a result of the casualties incurred by the army, British military command sought additional manpower and once again the issue of conscription was raised. The War Cabinet concluded that an extra 555,000 men in Great Britain and 150,000 in Ireland would be eligible for war service should they extend the terms of the Military Service Act.[93] In 1917, David Lloyd George, Prime Minister of the British Coalition Government, had refused to accede to demands from members of his War Cabinet to conscript the Irish. Lloyd George expressed his concerns about the concept of Irish conscription in a letter to Lord Riddell, liaison between the British government and press, arguing that it would cause scenes in the House of Commons, a possible rupture with America and serious dissatisfaction in Canada, Australia and South Africa. They would say, he claimed, 'you are fighting for the freedom of nationalities. What right have you to take this little nation by the ears and drag it into the war against its will'?[94]

Given the need for manpower in 1918, however, Lloyd George reneged and in April, extended conscription to Ireland. The decision to extend conscription to Ireland caused outrage among sections of the Irish population, including the Sinn Féin political party.[95] On 18 April 1918, Sinn Féin held a conference in the Mansion House, Dublin, and pledged to oppose conscription.[96] As a result, public support for Sinn Féin grew. The anti-conscription reaction was severe. Lord French, appointed as Ireland's Lord Lieutenant in May 1918, requested additional British Army troops in Ireland to try to control public aggression and disorder.[97] Due to the severity of the Irish reaction, the implementation of conscription in Ireland was continuously delayed. In France, the German offensive failed by July, and the Allies counter-attacked successfully at the Second Battle of the Marne and the Hundred Days Offensive. Consequently, conscription was never implemented in Ireland.

Against the backdrop of the increasing anti-war sentiment in Ireland, medical educational institutions remained supportive of the British war effort. In June 1918, the president of the Royal College of Physicians of Ireland, in a letter to Sir John Denton Pinkstone French, Lord Lieutenant General and General Governor of Ireland, reaffirmed the College's position on the war:

> We welcome the opportunity of expressing to you our unwavering attachment to the empire and our confidence in the ultimate triumph of the cause for which our people and our allies are fighting ... We desire to assure your excellency of our readiness to afford to his majesty and to his government as hearty assistance in this time of the empire's peril and to express again our loyalty to his throne.[98]

Yet by 1918, Irish medical recruitment rates had stalled and less than two per cent of those sampled enlisted in the RAMC in that year (Fig. 2.1). This was a dramatic drop from enlistment figures in the previous years. It was also in direct contrast to the recruitment patterns of regular Irish men enlisting in the combat forces of the British Army, whose recruitment levels increased in early 1918 and from August to November.[99] Approximately fifty-six per cent of non-medical Irish personnel enlisting in those periods joined the Royal Air Force, which, as Jeffery posits, attracted young men with labouring and technical opportunities.[100] Similarly, the Irish Medical War Committee focused its 1918 recruitment campaign entirely on securing as many young medical personnel from medical schools, promoting the corps as an advantageous career option. As late as October 1918, the Irish Committee launched a fresh appeal in association with the medical educational institutions and the licencing bodies, urging young doctors, particularly recently qualified graduates, to enrol. In the appeal, published in the *British Medical Journal*, the committee declared that 'apart altogether from the appeal which is made to them from the wounded, those who help will have the opportunities of great experience and of laying the foundations of a successful career'.[101] However, given the enlistment rates in 1918, their appeal was clearly not successful.

While it is possible that the political situation in Ireland had a bearing on enlistment rates in 1918, it is more likely that by the closing stages of war, Ireland's medical profession was simply stretched to the limit. Throughout 1917 and 1918, the Central Medical War Committee informed Alfred Keogh and the Ministry of National Service that they had run out of available medical manpower for the army in Britain.[102] A similar situation existed in Ireland. In February 1918, R. Marlay Blake, President of the Irish Medical Association, argued that the Irish medical profession had sent more men to the war 'in proportion to our numbers than did the profession in England'.[103] By June 1918, the Royal College of Physicians of Ireland reported that 'of those that had obtained the license of the college since the outbreak of the war, some ninety per cent have entered either the naval or military service'.[104] Therefore, by the closing stages of war, Ireland had contributed a considerable proportion of its medical personnel to the British Army and the removal of more was impracticable given the growing detrimental effect of war on domestic medical provision.

## CONCLUSION

From 1914 to 1918, approximately half of Ireland's doctors participated in the First World War. The enlistment rate of Irish doctors was comparable to that of British medics but differed from those of fellow Irishmen entering into the combat forces of the army. Moreover, the Irish Medical War Committee was central to securing high rates of recruitment of doctors in Ireland. From 1915 onwards, the committee managed medical recruitment and through its dealings with the LGBI, ensured that Irish doctors continued to enlist. While it is posited here that the Easter Rising had little effect on medical recruitment, it is clear that the overriding uneasy political situation in Ireland ultimately disrupted the enlistment of doctors into the British Army medical services. Given the disruptive actions of several boards of guardians regarding medical appointments, it can be persuasively argued that medical recruitment during the First World War suffered due to the guardians' wider campaign of antagonism towards the LGBI. By cancelling the appointments of locums and expressing open hostility towards the LGBI's strict adherence to professional protectionist agendas, these guardians discouraged Irish doctors from enlisting and, as we will see in a later chapter, caused distress for medical officers who had already joined and feared for their jobs at home. This is not to say that the guardians' actions wholly derailed wartime medical recruitment in Ireland. On the contrary, medical recruitment in Ireland, at least in the early years of the war, must be considered a success.

By the latter stages of war, however, the Irish medical profession was stretched and as many Irish medical professionals had enlisted into the British Army medical services as was possible. While Winter has argued that this did not cause a crisis in the provision of healthcare to civilians in Britain, the evidence examined here indicates that this was not the case in Ireland. The enlistment of doctors into the army harmed aspects of medical provision for Irish civilians. Certain regions, especially rural areas, throughout Ireland experienced a shortage of doctors, and some towns had no doctors at all. The failure of the LGBI to compromise with guardians and reach agreements on wartime employment regulations for medical officers not only threatened medical recruitment into the British Army but also accentuated the lack of availability of medical care to the Irish rural population during wartime.

## NOTES

1. Henry Jellett to the board of the Rotunda Hospital, 28 November 1914 (RCPI, Kirkpatrick collection, TCPK/6/5/14).
2. Arthur Sloggett to Dean and Registrar of the RCPI, 1 August 1914 (RCPI, RCPI papers, RCPI/2/3/3/14).
3. Director General of Royal Navy to Dean and Registrar of the RCPI, 30 July 1914 (RCPI, RCPI papers, RCPI/2/3/3/14).
4. RCPI Clerk to Arthur Sloggett, 4 August 1914 (RCPI, RCPI papers, RCPI/2/3/3/14).

5. Henry Jellett to the board of Rotunda Hospital, 28 November 1914 (RCPI, Kirkpatrick collection, TCPK/6/5/14).
6. Whitehead, *Doctors in the Great War*, pp. 60–90; Winter, *The Great War*, pp. 154–172.
7. Whitehead, *Doctors in the Great War*, p. 54.
8. Harrison, *The medical war*, p. 18.
9. Ryan, *Haig's* medical officer, p. 25.
10. Harrison, *The medical war*, p. 19.
11. *Irish Times*, 6 August 1914.
12. Anon., 'Ireland' in *British Medical Journal*, 2798, no. 2 (1914), p. 346.
13. This sample has been compiled from several sources including newspapers, such as the *Irish Times*, Irish Independent, *Freeman's Journal*. Further sources included the Kirkpatrick Index (Royal College of Physicians of Ireland [Hereafter RCPI], TPCK/5/3); *War list and roll of honour of the National University of Ireland* (Dublin, 1919); *Ireland's memorial records, 1914–18: Being the names of Irishmen who fell in the Great European War* (Dublin, 1923); *British Medical Journal*, 1880–1945; William Drew, William Johnston and Alfred Peterkin, *Commissioned officers in the medical services of the British Army, 1660–1960* (London: Wellcome Historical Medical Library, 1968).
14. A higher percentage of doctors enlisted in 1915 but 1915 was a twelve-month period. As per the sample: there was an average of 16 enlistments per month in 1915 and 32 per month in 1914 (August–December).
15. Callan, 'Voluntary recruiting for the British Army in Ireland', p. 49.
16. *Report on recruiting in Ireland* [Cd. 8168], H.C. 1916, xxxix, 525.
17. Bridget Hourican, 'Guest, Sir Ivor Churchill 1st Viscount Wimborne' in McGuire and Quinn (eds.), *Dictionary of Irish biography*, iv, 309.
18. Peter Gray and Olwen Purdue (eds.), *The Irish Lord Lieutenancy: c.1541–1922* (Dublin: University College Dublin Press, 2012).
19. *Report on Recruiting in Ireland*, pp. 1–4; Callan, 'Voluntary recruiting for the British Army in Ireland', p. 167.
20. Winter, *The Great War*, p. 155.
21. Anon., 'Medical War Committee' in *British Medical Journal*, 28231, no. 1 (1915), p. 268.
22. Anon., 'Central Medical War Committee' in *British Medical Journal*, 2865, no. 2 (1915), p. 785.
23. For full list of CMWC members, see Appendix A: Table A.2.
24. Anon., 'Thomas Hennessy' in *British Medical Journal*, 3914, no. 1 (1936), p. 87.
25. CMWC minute book, 9 August 1916 (TNA, MH 47/162).
26. For full list of IMWC members, see Appendix A: Table A.3.
27. Anon., 'Recruiting for the Naval and Military Medical Services' in *British Medical Journal*, 2877, no. 1 (1916), p. 617.

28. Whitehead, *Doctors in the Great War*, p. 45.
29. Virginia Crossman, *Poverty and the poor law in Ireland, 1850–1914* (Liverpool: Liverpool University Press, 2013), p. 1. Also see Ronald D. Cassell, *Medical charities, medical politics: The Irish dispensary system and the poor law, 1836–1872* (London: Royal Historical Society, 1997), pp. 78–108.
30. Catherine Cox, 'Health and welfare in Enniscorthy, 1850–1920' in Colm Toibin (ed.), *Enniscorthy: A history* (Wexford: Wexford County Council Public Service Library, 2010), p. 270.
31. Cox, 'Health and welfare', p. 271.
32. Anon., 'Irish Medical War Committee' in *British Medical Journal*, 2877, no. 1 (1916), p. 289.
33. For more information on Local Government in Ireland, see Mary E. Daly, *The buffer state: The historical roots of the Department of the Environment* (Dublin: Institute of Public Administration, 1997); Mary E. Daly (ed.), *County and town: One hundred years of local government in Ireland* (Dublin: Institute of Public Administration, 2001).
34. Thomas Hennessy, 'Irish Medical War Committee' in *British Medical Journal*, 2864, no. 2 (1915), p. 764.
35. 'R. (Lismore Guardians) v The Local Government Board (1)', King's Bench Division minutes, www.justis.com, accessed 12 May 2012.
36. *The Irish Times*, 7 April 1917.
37. *Freeman's Journal*, 1 April 1915.
38. Benson, 'The effect of war on the medical profession', p. 85.
39. Benson, 'The effect of war on the medical profession', p. 85.
40. Jeffery, *Ireland and the Great War*, p. 10.
41. Callan, 'British Recruitment in Ireland', p. 49.
42. Fitzpatrick, 'The logic of collective sacrifice', p. 1021.
43. Jeffery, *Ireland and the Great War*, p. 8.
44. Michael Taaffe, *Those days are gone away* (London: Hutchinson, 1959), p. 181.
45. Taaffe, *Those Days*, p. 181.
46. Terrence Denman, *Ireland's unknown soldiers: The 16th Division in the Great War* (Dublin: Irish Academic Press, 1992), pp. 43–60.
47. Central Medical War Committeee (Hereafter CMWC) minute book, 9 August 1916 (TNA, MH 47/162).
48. Stafford Adye-Curran (RCPI, Kirkpatrick Index, TPCK/5/3).
49. Diaries of Stafford Adye-Curran, 5 April 1915 (National Library of Ireland [Hereafter NLI], MS 34,393).
50. *Irish Times*, 28 September 1915.
51. *Irish Times*, 27 November 1915.
52. *Irish Times*, 21 December 1916.

53. *Belfast Newsletter*, 24 May 1915; *Medical Directory* 1921.
54. Winter, *The Great War*, p. 171.
55. Laura Kelly, *Irish women in medicine, c.1880s–1920s: Origins, education and careers* (Manchester: Manchester University Press, 2012), pp. 135–158.
56. Charles M. Benson, 'The effect of war on the medical profession' in *Dublin Journal of Medical Science*, Cxli (1916), p. 85.
57. Winter, *The Great War*, p. 170.
58. Captain T.F., 'The future of the medical profession' in *British Medical Journal*, 2925, no. 1 (1917), p. 86.
59. Winter, *The Great War*, p. 160.
60. *Irish Times*, 13 April 1915.
61. *Irish Times*, 13 April 1915.
62. *Irish Times*, 13 April 1915.
63. *Irish Times*, 9 June 1915.
64. *Irish Independent*, 2 November 1916.
65. *Freeman's Journal*, 18 January 1916.
66. *Irish Times*, 21 December 1916.
67. Anon., 'Medical recruiting' in *British Medical Journal*, 2875, no. 1 (1916), p. 214.
68. *Coventry Standard*, 3 March 1916.
69. *Coventry Standard*, 3 March 1916.
70. *Irish Independent*, 11 January 1918.
71. 'R. (Lismore Guardians) v The Local Government Board (1)', King's Bench Division Minutes, www.justis.com, accessed 12 May 2012. There were exceptions. Medical officers of military age who were exempt from war service due to health reasons were eligible for employment in the unions. In March 1918, for example, Dr. D. A. MacErlean applied for a dispensary post in the North Dublin Union and requested Dr. John O'Donnell, physician at the Mater Hospital, to inform the North Dublin Guardians that he (MacErlean) had myocardial troubles and a 'very irregular heart, and also suffered from pronounced amenia … and is utterly unfit for anything bordering on military service' so that he could secure the role. For more see North Dublin Union Board of Guardians minute book, 18 March 1918 (National Archives of Ireland [Hereafter NAI], MFGS 49/130).
72. Anon., 'Irish Medical War Committee' in *British Medical Journal*, 2879, no. 1 (1916), p. 359; Anon., 'Poor law medical officers on military service' in *British Medical Journal*, 2860, no. 2 (1915), p. 622.
73. Virginia Crossman, *Politics, pauperism and power in late nineteenth-century Ireland* (Manchester: Manchester University Press, 2006), p. 39.

74. William L. Feingold, 'The tenant's movement to capture the Irish Poor Law boards, 1877–1886' in *Albion: A Quarterly Journal Concerned with British Studies 7*, no. 3 (1975), p. 225.

75. Crossman, *Politics, pauperism and power*, p. 36.

76. Crossman, *Politics, pauperism and power*, p. 47.

77. *Connaught Telegraph*, 18 March 1916.

78. *Connaught Telegraph*, 18 March 1916.

79. *Connaught Telegraph*, 18 March 1916.

80. *Kerry Sentinel*, 27 September 1916.

81. The Lismore Board of guardians had shown increasing support for the nationalist cause in the past. See Crossman, *Politics, pauperism and power*, p. 52.

82. *Irish Examiner*, 6 July 1915; *Munster Express*, 15 February 1919; *Irish Examiner*, 20 January 1919.

83. 'R. (Lismore Guardians) v The Local Government Board (1)', King's Bench Division Minutes, www.justis.com, accessed 12 May 2012.

84. 'R. (Lismore Guardians) v The Local Government Board (1)', King's Bench Division Minutes, www.justis.com, accessed 12 May 2012.

85. 'R. (Lismore Guardians) v The Local Government Board (1)', King's Bench Division Minutes, www.justis.com, accessed 12 May 2012.

86. South Dublin Union Board of Guardians minute book, 30 May 1917 (NAI, MFGS 49/89).

87. According to comparison of enlistment sources and *Medical Directory*, 1914–1918; It is important to note here that medical directories have been criticised for being unreliable at times; the directories contain information compiled from returns submitted by practitioners throughout Ireland. Their accuracy therefore relied on the accuracy of the records submitted by the doctors themselves. According to Cox a significant proportion of the physicians and surgeons did not return their details, particularly during times of national crisis, like the Great Famine, and consequently those who compiled the data sought the information from elsewhere. See Catherine Cox, 'The medical marketplace and medical tradition in nineteenth-century Ireland' in Ronnie Moore and Stuart McClean (eds.), *Folk healing and health care practices in Britain and Ireland: Stethoscopes, wands and crystals* (Oxford, 2010), p. 62. While twentieth-century directories are more reliable, those created during the war years do note that some information is missing. To minimise this problem, where possible, the medical directories (1914–1918) have been supplemented by medical directories released in the years after the war, which were more complete, and by the Kirkpatrick Index.

88. Winter, *The Great War*, p. 155.

89. Anon., 'Ireland' in *British Medical Journal*, 2966, no. 2 (1917), p. 602.

90. *Connaught Telegraph*, 18 March 1916.
91. *The Irish Times*, 19 February. 1917.
92. William Mulligan, *The Great War for peace* (New Haven: Yale University Press, 2014), p. 253.
93. Hennessy, *Dividing Ireland*, p. 220.
94. George A. Riddell, *Lord Riddell's war diary, 1914–18* cited in Alan J. Ward, 'Lloyd George and the 1918 conscription crisis' in *The Historical Journal* 17, no. 1 (1974), p. 109.
95. Ward, 'Lloyd George', p. 115.
96. Hennessy, *Dividing Ireland*, p. 221.
97. Ward, 'Lloyd George', p. 117.
98. President of the RCPI to the Lord Lieutenant General and General Governor of Ireland, 7 June 1918 (RCPI, RCPI collection, RCPI/2/3/3/14, RCPI).
99. The number of Irish recruits who enlisted from February 1918–August 1918 was 5812 while 9845 enlisted from August 1918–11 November 1918 (3 and a half months). See Callan, 'British recruitment in Ireland', p. 49; Jeffery, *Ireland and the Great War*, p. 7.
100. Jeffery, *Ireland and the Great War*, p. 7.
101. Anon., 'Immediate need of doctors for the army' in *British Medical Journal*, 3015, no. 2 (1918), p. 417.
102. CMWC minute book, 26 January 1917 (TNA, MH 47/162).
103. Letter from R. Marlay Blake to the editor, *Irish Independent*, 6 February 1918.
104. President of the RCPI to the Lord Lieutenant General and General Governor of Ireland, 7 June 1918 (RCPI, RCPI collection, RCPI/2/3/3/14, RCPI).

# CHAPTER 3

# Irish Medical Personnel: Motivations and Wartime Experiences, 1914–1918

'[There is] nothing to do in the way of work. A child could do all there is to be done'.[1]

By the end of 1914, heads of universities throughout Ireland were publicly praising their former medical students for enlisting in the RAMC. On 27 November 1914, Justice Madden, vice-chancellor of the senate of TCD, contended that for 'no class of students has the call of duty been more fully recognised than by students of the School of Physic. Since the war began, a large number of young medical graduates have received temporary commissions'.[2] Yet these genres of speeches seldom offered real insight into the reasons for Irish doctors' enlistment. This chapter is concerned with the doctors' motivations to participate in the First World War and it will consider whether these altered over the course of the conflict. Several studies have examined the reasons for Irish medical migration in the nineteenth and twentieth centuries. Jones has analysed Irish medical migration between 1860 and 1905, while Steven O'Connor has examined principal causes of Irish medical migration during the 1930s and 1940s. Both have argued that overcrowding in the Irish medical profession encouraged the migration of Irish doctors to elsewhere and their subsequent enlistment in the British Army.[3]

The motivations behind Irish medical involvement in the First World War have yet to be uncovered. For Irish soldiers—non-medical personnel—Fitzpatrick and Jeffery have identified several push and pull factors

© The Author(s) 2019
D. Durnin, *The Irish Medical Profession and the First World War*,
Medicine and Biomedical Sciences in Modern History,
https://doi.org/10.1007/978-3-030-17959-5_3

that encouraged their enlistments into the military during the conflict.[4] Fitzpatrick, for example, has argued that peer pressure was instrumental and that those belonging to militias, fraternities and sporting clubs were susceptible to collective pressures that encouraged them to enlist.[5] Jeffery posits that a belief in the just cause of the war prompted enlistment.[6] This chapter will consider whether Irish doctors enlisted for similar reasons or were motivated by factors associated more explicitly with the medical profession.

Moreover, this chapter will examine the social backgrounds of Irish doctors who served with the RAMC during the First World War. It will analyse several categories, including the age, marital status and education of doctors to explore whether there were links between their background and motivations for participating in the war. The absence of similar studies for other national medical contingents makes it is impossible to compare the social profile of Irish doctors with their English, Scottish or Welsh counterparts. Marcus Ackroyd, Laurence Brockliss, Michael Moss, Kate Retford and John Stevenson, however, have meticulously detailed the social profile of Irish doctors who enlisted in the British Army between 1790 and 1850 and served in the Napoleonic and Boer Wars.[7] To explore continuities, this chapter will compare, where possible, the social profile of Ireland's First World War doctors to their predecessors.

While studies on the backgrounds of First World War medical participants are scarce, several historians have detailed the roles and experiences of British doctors in the conflict. For instance, Whitehead has analysed the role of doctors on the battlefields of the Western Front while Harrison has expertly examined the development of military medicine and the structures the RAMC employed to ensure efficiency and success in the treatment of wounded soldiers.[8] The second section of this chapter is concerned specifically with the roles and experiences of Irish medical personnel—doctors and nurses—within the British Army's First World War 'medical machine', examining the Field Ambulance (FA) divisions, Casualty Clearing Stations (CCS) and war hospitals.[9] Other studies have argued that military medical command assigned contingents of medics to especially onerous tasks because of their nationality.[10] This chapter will ask whether Irish medical personnel's wartime experiences differed in comparison to their English, Scottish and Welsh colleagues.[11] It will additionally attempt to investigate whether the outbreak of the armed insurrection against British rule in Ireland in 1916 affected these experiences.

## Motivations

Dr. J. P. Lynch, a County Cork native and Captain in the RAMC, was a career army medic who had joined the British Army medical services in 1904. He noted feelings of 'supressed excitement' among colleagues at his local barracks in Canterbury, England, as they mobilised for despatch in August 1914.[12] Lynch was among the thirty-five per cent of Irish doctors who served in the First World War that had already enlisted in the British Army prior to the outbreak of conflict (Fig. 2.1). The evidence suggests that pre-war recruits, such as Lynch, shared similar motivations for enlisting into the British Army medical services as those who enlisted from 1914 to 1918 to serve solely for the duration of the war.

Both pre-war and wartime recruits enlisted into the RAMC to earn a wage. Jones has argued that Britain's Army medical services offered viable employment prospects to members of the Irish medical profession.[13] To understand the financial attraction of the British army to the Irish doctor, it is important to appreciate the state of the medical profession in Ireland and Britain in the years prior to the First World War. From the early nineteenth century, middle-class men became increasingly attracted to the medical profession and the numbers entering medical schools throughout Britain and Ireland rose to unprecedented levels as the century progressed.[14] During this period, Ireland's reputation as a significant centre of medical education increased. In his study of the Catholic University Medical School, F. O. C. Meenan claimed that for a brief phase during the middle years of the nineteenth century 'Dublin was the leading centre of world medicine'.[15] While this is debatable, there is no doubt that the popularity of medical education in Ireland was growing. An 1878 student guide to the medical profession stated that 'if the number of students be considered, the medical school of Dublin is larger than that of London, or indeed any other town of the United Kingdom'.[16]

Due to the popularity of Ireland's medical courses, the number of qualified doctors in search of work increased. Many found employment in hospital appointments, general practice and poor law posts. However, there were simply insufficient opportunities in Ireland to cater for the streams of medical graduates emerging from Ireland's educational institutions and the Irish medical profession was severely overcrowded.[17] As Jones has suggested, Ireland's medical schools were thus primarily exporting institutions that produced more graduates than could be employed in Ireland.[18] Large numbers of Irish doctors thus moved abroad to earn a living and among them were those who sought commissions in the British Army medical services.

Recently qualified medical graduates rather than high-earning general practitioners enlisted into the RAMC for the salary. An 1879 report on pay and conditions in the Army medical services determined that an assistant surgeon in the forces earned £200 per annum that would increase incrementally to *c.* £500 per annum after fifteen years. A pension and sizeable payment, sufficient to allow men to establish a private practice, was also available on retirement.[19] By 4 August 1914, the RAMC had improved their remuneration package and a doctor on active service received around £400 a year and a uniform allowance.[20] Those who enlisted on temporary wartime commissions joined on a twelve-month contract, or until the war had ended, whichever occurred first. Commissions were often renewed over the course of the war. While the rate of pay for appointments in the medical divisions of the British Army had improved marginally in the decade before the war, it was mediocre when compared to the incomes of successful general practitioners. A newly qualified medical graduate could expect to earn an income of £280–£360 from private practice and other MO work at the start of their careers while a more established general practitioner was regularly earning £800–£1000 a year.[21] Well-established general practitioners and those in hospital posts could not consider the War Office's rate of pay sufficient compensation for income lost from their regular civilian posts and practices.

In the early months of war, some Irish doctors in state-funded appointments—poor law dispensary, workhouse and lunatic asylum MOs—who had not established a successful private practice benefited financially from enlistment. During this time, the poor law MOs who joined the RAMC retained full pay from their dispensary posts while at war. In April 1915, for instance, Dr. McCarthy, Glengarriff dispensary MO, applied to Bantry Board of Guardians in County Cork for temporary leave of absence to serve in the RAMC. B. O'Connor, temporary chairman of the board, sanctioned his leave. However, J. Gilhooly, another guardian, objected because McCarthy would continue to receive a full wage during his absence, even though he was 'not providing any medical service to the ratepayers of Glengarriff District'. After much deliberation, the board decided to seek remuneration from the LGBI to pay a substitute MO and McCarthy retained his whole salary.[22]

McCarthy thus received two incomes during his wartime service—one from the RAMC and another from the Bantry Board of Guardians. From late 1915 onwards, it was common for departing doctors retain a portion of their state salary—usually half—which they received in addition to their RAMC pay.[23] Irish nurses who were employed in state posts also departed on similar terms. The governors of the House of Industry Hospitals agreed to pay Edith Holden, the hospitals' matron, £80 per annum—a portion of her salary—while she served in the war.[24] Holden noted that the salary given to her by the board, with the £75 she received from the War Office, would bring her total income to £155—'more than the £132 she was receiving before the war'.[25]

Debates regarding pay for those taking leave from their poor law posts to enlist were commonplace at guardians' meetings. In October 1915, an argument broke out at a meeting of the Limerick Board of Guardians when Dr. Joseph Humphreys, MO for Bridgestown dispensary district, requested twelve months leave from his position to enlist in the RAMC. Several members of the board immediately spoke out in Humphreys' favour, with Mr. McNamara declaring that 'that is pluck anyway' and Mr. Quilligan noting that Humphreys was doing his 'part as a man'.[26] These proposed that Humphreys receive half his MO salary during his leave. Others objected to this, including P. Bourke who argued that Humphreys was 'going to benefit himself. That was no patriotism' and he should only enlist if he was doing so at his own expense, without remuneration from his MO position.[27] A vote was conducted and thirty-one guardians voted in favour of Humphrey receiving a salary, while Bourke, along with twenty-one others, voted against. Following the vote, Mr. Donnellan, a member of the board, addressed those who had voted against as 'Sinn Féiners' and arguments erupted throughout the room. In a closing address to the Board, Dr. Humphreys noted that following his return from war, 'he would treat every one of those who voted against him the same way that as they treated their country'.[28]

While the RAMC salary certainly enticed medical personnel to participate in the war, others enlisted even though it reduced their annual income. Fitzpatrick and Jeffery have both emphasised that influences other than economic motivation encouraged Irish enlistment into the British Army.[29] Fitzpatrick, in particular, has argued that the 'logic of economic rationality' cannot fully account for the recruitment of Irish men into British Army combat regiments.[30] The same was true for Irish doctors. In 1916, for example, three out of the four poor law MOs in the

Abbeyleix Union of Queen's County enlisted and agreed to relinquish their salaries as poor law MOs for the duration of their wartime service.[31] Some general practitioners also volunteered their services despite having well-established private practices in cities and rural districts. In December 1915, for instance, Dr. John O'Boyle enlisted in the RAMC for the duration of the war, leaving his 'extremely remunerative' private practice in Ballina, County Mayo.[32] It is thus essential to examine the non-economic factors that motivated Irish doctors to enlist in the RAMC.

Patriotic fervour certainly propelled Irish doctors to enlist. Phillip Orr has suggested that Irish men entered the British Army in a 'surge of naive patriotism'.[33] Recruiting committees attempted to stir up feelings of patriotism among the Irish population to encourage enlistments. In 1914, James Abraham, an Irish surgeon who enlisted, recalled that 'posters of Kitchener stared me in the face everywhere, pointing with an exaggerated hand, saying: "your King and country need you"'.[34] Medical recruitment committees and key figures in medical education emphasised patriotic duty in their pleas for volunteers. In March 1915, Frederick Conway Dwyer, RCSI President and IMWC member, in an address at an RCSI licencing ceremony, noted that his usual task of offering career advice to graduates was much easier that year:

> Graduates should enter as speedily as possible the Royal Army Medical Corps to place their professional skill and knowledge at the disposal of their King and country. Of the absolute propriety and necessity of that choice from every point of view there can be no question. In giving their services to the Empire in her hour of supremest need they were fulfilling the paramount duty of every citizen.[35]

According to Dwyer, it was the duty of Irish doctors, as citizens of the British Empire, to involve themselves in the war effort. IMWC references to doctors' patriotism continued throughout the war. In December 1916, Dr. Maurice Hayes, IMWC secretary, defended Irish doctors' honour after an article in the *Irish Times* questioned medical men's patriotism; the author of the article stated, 'though the doctors have a splendid record in this war, patriotism has not been universal'.[36] In response, Hayes' argued '[these statements] so far as they apply to Irish doctors individually and collectively, are not only without foundation, but they are a stigma on their patriotism and integrity'.[37] Boards of guardians also regularly referred to volunteer doctors' patriotic nature when permitting their MOs to leave their posts to participate in the war. In 1915, the Bantry Board of Guardians, after approving Dr. McCarthy's leave of absence, congratulated him on 'his spirit of patriotism and loyalty to the cause of the empire, and hoped his good example would be numerously followed'.[38]

In his study of the enlistment of Irish officers into the British forces from 1922 to 1945, O'Connor has argued that Irish doctors often enlisted during this period because of family links to the services.[39] This was also evident throughout the First World War. Family tradition encouraged medical personnel into the British Army to serve in the conflict. Doctors whose relatives—father, uncle or brother—had at some point served in the British Army medical services often followed their example. William Cherry, a graduate of the RCSI who enlisted in the British Army medical services in 1902, served in the war as Fleet Surgeon in the Royal Navy. His father, William Cherry Sr. had had a distinguished career in the British Army medical services during the nineteenth century, rising to the rank of Deputy Surgeon General prior to his retirement in 1887.[40] In several cases, Irish families had more than one member serving in the RAMC during the First World War. In 1914, John O'Connell, a County Kerry native, followed his father David into service in the RAMC. Lieutenant Colonel David O'Connell outlived his son following John's death in September 1914 during the First Battle of Aisne. In 1915, Frederick Carson from County Antrim entered the RAMC after his brother James, a captain in the corps, died during fighting in Egypt. Two of his other brothers were also in the British Army medical services.[41]

Recruiters exploited feelings of moral compulsion that manifested among some sections of the Irish population as a consequence of the violent nature of the war.[42] This encouraged the Irish medical profession to enlist. For instance, members of the IMWC often urged colleagues at medical conferences and graduation ceremonies to enlist because of the suffering caused by the violent conflict:

> bearing in mind the ready response which its former appeals have received, and acknowledging the valuable service which the Irish doctors have hitherto rendered in the war, the committee believes that this appeal will not be made in vain and that all the call of suffering humanity will find a ready response from Irish medical men, whose sympathy and generous self-sacrifice in alleviation of suffering have become traditional ... this is an appeal to them from the wounded.[43]

Reports from troops and medics near the frontlines supported the IMWC's rhetoric. In their letters and postcards home, many of those in the British Army recounted stories of violent German atrocities. A. Doran, an Irishman enlisted in the RAMC and based in France, wrote a postcard to his family simply stating 'they shelled us out of the Brewery. They have no respect for the Red Cross flag, the dirty devils'.[44] On 25 June 1915, shortly after a series of setbacks effecting British morale, including the sinking of the *Lusitania* and the battles of Krithia, Stafford Adye-Curran noted in his journal that 'it is pure unadulterated cold blooded murder on both sides. But ours is certainly justified as goodness knows the men have had just cause'.[45]

Economic motivation, patriotism and moral justification was evident in both the enlistment of Irishmen into the combat forces of the British Army and doctors into the RAMC. However, there were also motivational factors which were solely related to members of the medical profession. In the early months of the war, senior doctors contended that it was the responsibility of the medical profession to participate in the conflict. On 3 December 1914, Thomas E. Gordon, surgeon to the Adelaide Hospital, Dublin, argued in an address delivered to the student's union of the RCSI that

> If it were my duty to urge you to learn the use of the rifle and bayonet I should dwell on a more stirring motive still – the defence of our homes, our women, our children, and all else we hold dear, against a savage and cruel barbarism. My message for you tonight is different … For you there is a call to join a band of men to whom are entrusted the highest use of science; whose duty it is, not to destroy life, but if possible, to save it, to relieve the suffering and to heal the wounded … With the soldier you are called to a work of self-sacrifice – it may be to acts of heroism; you must share with him the dangers of battle, but unlike him, you must in your work, see no difference between friend and foe; for you the only enemies are disease and pain and death; for you it is to "love your enemies"; for you it is indeed to fight – but under the banner of the Prince of Peace.[46]

As Gordon's speech demonstrates, the rhetoric used by medical men in favour of wartime participation emphasised that it was a doctor's responsibility to enlist given their professional skill. In his 1915 address to the RCSI, Dwyer reiterated a similar message. He argued that doctors were 'fortunate enough to be in the position of performing their duty with consciousness of being equipped with a technical professional skill which enormously enhances the value of their services'.[47]

Peer pressure was influential in promoting this responsibility among doctors and encouraged self-mobilisation in the medical profession. Horne has defined self-mobilisation in wartime as the mobilisation of society without state coercion. It was, he argues, particularly evident among all kinds of social groups and institutions in Britain, France and Germany during the first two years of war.[48] Certainly, the Irish medical profession was characterised by a high degree of voluntary self-mobilisation during the conflict as doctors formed the IMWC and enlisted without compulsion. An important element of self-mobilisation among the professions was the consistent peer pressure, stemming primarily from senior figures, which sustained enlistment rates. Friends and educational mentors successfully encouraged Ireland's medical men to join.[49] Medical personnel also regularly discussed participation in the war among themselves at events. At their 1915 annual general meeting, members of the Ulster Medical Society discussed the wartime roles of nineteen of their members who had enlisted to serve in the war.[50] Several other societies and educational institutions such as the Biological Society of Ireland and the RCPI organised conferences to discuss the theme of war and medicine.[51] On 1 November 1916, during the brutal closing stages of the Battle of the Somme, the Biological Society of the RCSI dedicated their opening meeting to a discussion of the role of members of the Irish medical profession in the First World War. Captain Gillman Moorhead, an Irish TCD graduate, addressed the meeting and detailed his experiences of working in the base hospital in Alexandria—'the tropical heat of the summer months and the abundance of flies made conditions especially trying'. He encouraged more Irish doctors to get involved.[52] Surgeon General Richard Ford, Deputy Director of Medical Services, RAMC Irish Command, also in attendance, commended the society's work and actively encouraged those in attendance to follow the example that had been set.[53]

Collective pressure, of course, was not confined to universities, societies or the workplace. Ireland's doctors, surgeons and physicians socialised together. In 1915 several members of a Masonic Lodge in County Armagh volunteered together for service in the RAMC.[54] Doctors also participated together in various sporting associations throughout the country. Fitzpatrick has suggested that recruitment committees were well aware of the 'power of the sporting motif' and attempted to enlist a sports club's entire contingent of members.[55] In his study of the role of Irish barristers in the First World War, Anthony Quinn has argued that glory on the sports field was emulated on the battlefield and thus it was logical for recruiters to target sports teams to secure men.[56] Irish doctors were heavily involved in local and national sports teams and their presence was frequent on the team sheets of several rugby football teams scattered throughout the country. As Quinn has noted, recruitment through Irish rugby networks was similar to recruitment in other parts of the United Kingdom where 'pals' battalions' were expressions of Edwardian civic pride.[57] During the First World War, the Dublin Hospital's Cup—a rugby tournament involving many of Dublin's hospitals including Sir Patrick Duns' and the Mater Misericordiae—was cancelled because the hospitals could not field teams due to their members' enlistment in the RAMC.[58]

From 1916 onwards, as the number of Irish medical recruits declined, the LGBI's strict adherence to its wartime employment regulations limited employment options for young Irish doctors and this motivated some to enlist in the RAMC. After the LGBI refused to sanction the temporary appointment of an MO of military age in the Boherbee dispensary district, the Kanturk Board of Guardians in County Cork accused the LGBI of using their regulations 'as a mean form of compulsion' to ensure that young doctors enlisted.[59] There was some merit to this accusation as in several cases, young doctors who had their temporary appointments to state posts vetoed by the LGBI subsequently enlisted in the RAMC. In March 1917, for instance, the LGBI refused to sanction the temporary appointment of Dr. Bernard Joseph O'Donnell as temporary MO to the Timoleague dispensary district, County Cork, because he was of military age. By May 1917, O'Donnell was serving with the RAMC in Mesopotamia.[60]

During the final months of the war, the IMWC continually highlighted the severity of the conflict's closing battles and their messages appealed to some of Irish doctors. On 3 October 1918, following the Battles of the Hindenburg Line—the Allied offensive attacks against German troops located at Rheims, Holnon and St. Quentin—the committee launched a final plea: 'owing to the heavy fighting which is at present taking place on the Western Front the resources of the RAMC have been taxed to the uttermost, and at the moment there is a very urgent need for young doctors at the front'.[61] As shown, however, only a small number of Irish doctors were encouraged to enlist as a consequence of these pleas.

## SOCIAL PROFILE

Irish doctors, thus, responded to several motivating factors encouraging them to enlist into the British Army medical services. Yet not all who applied were commissioned. During the opening months of the war, some British military leaders believed that victory would be swift and as a result, the War Office's recruitment plans were inadequate in many respects; volunteers in poor health and bad physical fitness were accepted into the army.[62] Early medical recruitment processes were also flawed. From August 1914 to the summer of 1915, the War Office focused almost solely on securing young doctors for the RAMC. In August 1914, the War Office informed the *British Medical Journal* that 'the immediate need of the army is the younger men who are prepared to enter the army and go anywhere they are sent' and that older doctors who wrote to the War Office seeking information on enlistment were unlikely to receive a response.[63] This resulted in cases of older doctors—thirty and above—presenting themselves to recruiting offices and being informed that it was unnecessary for them to enlist. In August 1914, Dr. James Abraham, living in Britain, visited his local war office to enlist. However, the enlistment officer informed Abraham that he was 'a bit old for us. You are over thirty and we really only want young newly qualified men to do dressings in the front line. We don't need Fellows of the College. You're too heavy guns for us. The war will be over by Christmas'.[64] In July 1915, the medical war committees altered the recruitment process and implemented their own regulations. From 1917 to Armistice Day on 11 November 1918, the committees eased these protocols as the severity of the war took its toll on RAMC numbers. The need for medical personnel began to outweigh concerns about suitability. During these three distinct periods of recruitment—August 1914 to October of 1915; November 1915 to February 1917 and April 1917 to Armistice Day—there were some slight alterations to the Irish medical recruit's profile.

For the most part, the War Office preferred to commission young, recent medical graduates as it filled the RAMC's ranks without sacrificing the medical provision for civilian society. Recent medical graduates' enlistment had minimal impact on civilian medical infrastructure when compared to the absence of more senior and well-established doctors. In the first months of war, the focus on youth encouraged medical students who had not yet graduated to enlist to dress wounds.[65] As early as December 1914, however, it became clear to those involved in the British war effort that the prediction of Lord Kitchener, Secretary of State for War, of a long-drawn-out conflict was accurate.[66] Consequently, Alfred Keogh decided that it would be best for medical students to enlist in the RAMC only after they had completed their studies. On 10 December 1914, Keogh noted in a letter to Donald MacAlister, General Medical Council President, that 'the senior student is best fulfilling his duty to the country by getting his degree and then joining the army'.[67] He encouraged medical students who had already enlisted to return and complete their studies, particularly those in the latter years of a medical degree who, in a rush for the front, had abandoned their studies to enlist, not only in the RAMC but also in the regular combat forces. Some of the students were not pleased. In March 1915, Charles Brennan, an RCSI student who enlisted in the RAMC, noted that

> on the 8[th] August last [I] was equipped and thought I would be called on immediately, but the war office changed their minds and alas, sent me home to get qualified. Since then I have been working hard and hope to get qualified in the minimum time next June (with luck). Also I have to sit near some dear old lady in a tram or theatre, who settles her spectacles on her nose, and looks at you, and sniffs, as much as to say "Are you funky?" I know at least a score of men in the same position, most of whom, including myself, have done their three or four years in an Officers Training Corps. They have to look at fellows in uniform and on duty who have never seen an Officers' Training Corps in their lives.[68]

In 1915, the IMWC took charge of recruitment, beginning the second period of medical recruitment in Ireland, and refused to commission medical students. Senior members of the Irish and British medical profession, those leading the IMWC and the CMWC, agreed with Alfred Keogh that it would be much more beneficial for the war effort to enlist medical students who had finished their studies prior to volunteering.[69] In most cases, Irish medical students completed their education and then immediately volunteered for the RAMC. To assist the recruitment process, Irish universities, including TCD, accelerated the conferring of degrees to senior medical students who had completed their exams and wished to join the RAMC.[70] Captain Eugene John McSwiney, from County Cork, was a typical example; McSwiney was educated at TCD and opted to remain after the outbreak of war. In 1915, he graduated with an M.B., a B.Ch. and a B.A.O following a quick conferral and immediately volunteered for the RAMC and served in France.[71]

On 19 November 1915, the CMWC created a table that detailed the profile of their ideal medical recruits—newly qualified doctors and junior MOs employed by a local authority (Table 3.1).

It is probable that the IMWC, as a subsidiary committee, adopted this table as a guide. By implementing these guidelines, the IMWC maintained the enlistment of young doctors into the British Army. The majority of volunteers accepted under the preferred candidate guideline were in their twenties—the most likely age group of newly qualified and junior medical men. As a result of this focus on securing young medical graduates, approximately forty per cent of Irish medical recruits were aged between twenty and twenty-nine (Fig. 3.1).

At the other end of the scale, doctors up to the age of forty-five could enlist in the British Army medical services according to the terms of the War Office recruitment regulations. The upper age limit for medical professionals enlisting in the services differed to their military counterparts; only those aged forty-one or below could join the combat forces.[72] According to an article in the *British Medical Journal*, the higher age limit for doctors was a direct result of the urgent need for medical expertise on the battlefields.[73] As Fig. 3.1 shows, however, approximately sixteen per cent of Irish medical wartime participants were above the maximum age limit. While the War Office normally refused

**Table 3.1**  Medical war committees' preferred candidate for service in the RAMC

| | |
|---|---|
| Single or married | All newly qualified men |
| | Junior medical men employed by local authorities |
| | Resident medical men at institutions |
| | Assistants and partners to general practitioners |
| Single | Chief TB Officers if not also MOs of health |
| | Men in single-handed private practices in cities |
| | Men replacing earlier volunteers |
| Married | Men in single-handed panel practices in cities |
| | Men in single-handed private practices in cities |
| Rural | Single men in single-handed private practices in rural areas |
| | Married men in single-handed private practices in rural areas |

*Source* CMWC Minutes, 19 November 1915, as cited in J. M. Winter, *The Great War*, p. 161

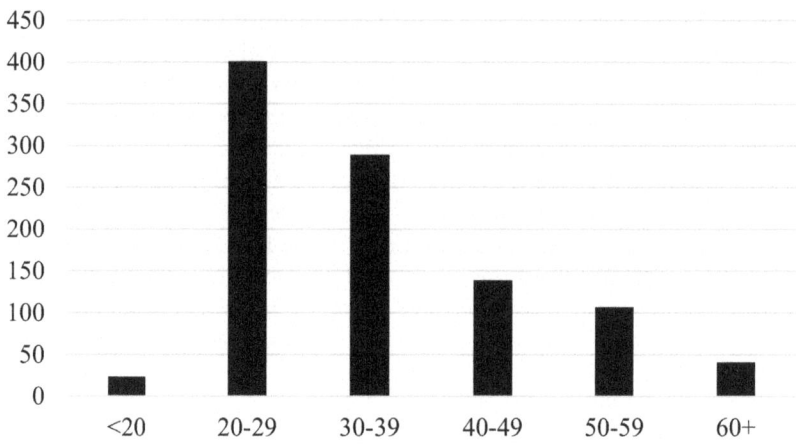

**Fig. 3.1** Age profile of Irish doctors and medical students who participated in the First World War (*Source* Database of Irish medical officers in British forces who served in the First World War—based on a sample of 1000 doctors)

to commission older men, some older doctors filled roles in Ireland and Britain as members of the RAMC's Home Hospital Reserve.[74] For instance, Dr. Robert Thompson, a fifty-three-year-old retired doctor from County Cork, volunteered for RAMC service immediately following the outbreak of hostilities. Thompson was posted to Tralee Barracks, in County Kerry, where he administered health checks and provided healthcare to new recruits in the camp.[75]

Many of the older doctors that enlisted had previously served with the British Army medical services and these men brought invaluable experience. Lieutenant Colonel John Riordan, aged fifty-eight from County Limerick, returned to the RAMC in 1914 having retired in 1903 following campaigns in Burma. Riordan secured a domestic role taking charge of the medical services at the Royal Irish Regiment Depot in Clonmel, County Tipperary.[76] Previous experience in specific battles or regiments often influenced the role assigned to older doctors throughout the First World War. In 1914, Lieutenant Colonel William Coates, a retired Indian Medical Services (IMSs) officer from Galway, re-enlisted in the RAMC. Due to his experience, RAMC authorities assigned Coates to serve in the specially constructed York Place Indian Hospital located in Brighton.[77] Caring for sick and wounded Indian soldiers was complex as it was essential to follow rules observing caste and religious differences that were crucial to maintaining soldiers' morale.[78] Thus, when the RAMC established an Indian hospital in Brighton, they recognised that it was important to staff it with medical men, even those over the maximum age for war service, who had experience dealing with Indian soldiers.

During the first period of recruitment, a number of Irish doctors over the age limit re-enlisted into the RAMC because of their administrative experience. Alfred Keogh was a prime example. In July 1914, Keogh, aged fifty-seven, retired from RAMC service but shortly after the outbreak of war, he returned to his role as Director General of the RAMC. His case was not unique. On 24 August 1914, the RAMC tasked Surgeon General William Donovan, who was aged sixty-four, with the role of Deputy Director of Medical Services of Embarkation at Southampton, England. Donovan, born in County Kerry and educated at TCD, previously served with the British Army medical services in the Afghan (1878–1880) and Boer Wars (1880–1881; 1899–1902), and obtained numerous honours and distinctions for his service.[79] At the outbreak of conflict, Southampton was chosen as the port of disembarkation in Britain for sick and wounded soldiers returning from France. Between 1914 and 1916, the RAMC transported over 600,000 wounded to Southampton docks.[80] Donovan administered the flow of wounded soldiers through the port and ensured that they were appropriately distributed to military hospitals throughout Britain and Ireland. Donovan secured this position because of previous experience and placing a role of such importance in the hands of a less experienced man may have jeopardised Britain's wartime casualty dispersal system.

Following the establishment of the IMWC in 1915, a decline in the enlistment rates of older Irish doctors was evident. It is likely that by that stage in war, those with valuable military medical experience had already re-enlisted. Yet the higher age limit appears to have been waived when the RAMC were most urgently in need of doctors. In April 1918, following the German Spring Offensive, the RAMC again sought older civilian doctors to supplement the shortfall in numbers and provide essential support. In this final recruitment period, Westminster passed the Military Service Act, which extended the maximum age for non-medical recruits to fifty-one.[81] While the Act did not apply to doctors, recruiting committees issued notices to reiterate and inform the medical profession that physicians and surgeons up to the age of

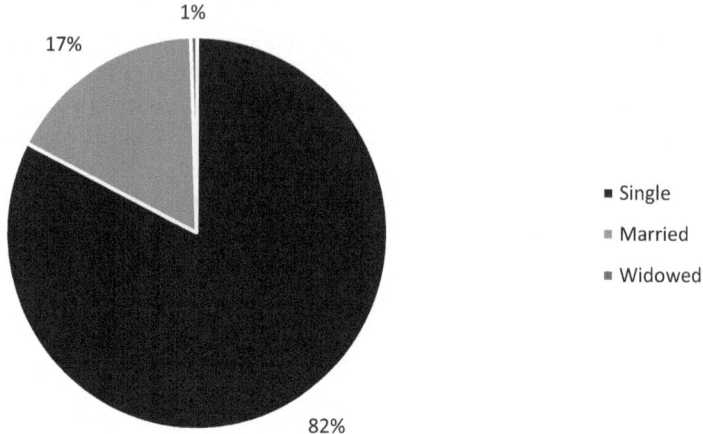

**Fig. 3.2** Marital status of Irish doctors who participated in the First World War (*Source* Database of Irish medical officers in British forces who served in the First World War—based on a sample of 400 doctors)

fifty-five could enlist in the British Army medical services on the condition that they serve in roles on the domestic front, including positions in the numerous military hospitals, wards and auxiliary units established throughout Ireland and Britain.

As well as focusing on recruits' age, the IMWC also considered their marital status. Eighty-two per cent of Irish doctors who enlisted in the British Army during the First World War were single and this pattern predates the establishment of the IMWC (Fig. 3.2). There are several explanations for this trend. Firstly, the rate of marriage in Ireland was lower than other European countries.[82] Secondly, the age of an Irish married couple was older than most other European nations with an average marriage age of twenty-nine for the women and thirty-three for the men.[83] Since the War Office and the RAMC sought young medical students and newly qualified graduates for RAMC commissions—who were usually below the age of twenty-nine—it was not surprising that the majority were single.

From 1915 to 1917, the IMWC's recruitment processes aided the continued enlistment of a high percentage of single medical men. The IMWC, similar to its British counterpart, preferred to enlist single doctors with minimal family commitments. Securing young, single males for service was not unique to medical recruitment as it was also common practice in the recruitment of men into combat forces. On 27 January 1916, the British Parliament passed the Military Service Act which formalised this preference; 'every male British subject who on August 15<sup>th</sup>, 1915, was ordinarily resident in Great Britain ... and was unmarried or was a widower without any child dependent on him [was compelled to enlist]'.[84] While the conscription clause detailed in this Act did not apply to either the medical profession or the Irish population, medical war committees maintained similar criteria in recruitment drives for the remainder of the conflict.

Of course, it was not possible to fulfil the requirements for manpower of the RAMC by relying wholly on the enlistment of single doctors. As Fig. 3.2 demonstrates, seventeen per cent of Irish doctors who enlisted in the British forces from 1914 to 1918 were married. Many of these were career army medics who had enlisted in the British Army medical or colonial services before 1914. While these men had experienced long spells of separation from their wives during previous assignments, they struggled emotionally during the First World War. Dr. J. P. Lynch acknowledged in his war diary that saying goodbye to his family immediately prior to his mobilisation was one of the most challenging moments of the entire conflict:

> the taxi came and Rosie [his wife] and I drove to the East station, it was an anxious drive, and I cannot describe how we felt while waiting in the station for the train, as the feeling of the unknown had taken possession of us, she did not know when she would see me again and I felt that I was about to part from her for a most indefinite period of time.[85]

Lynch was not alone. Other Irish doctors regularly noted their sadness at being parted from their wives in their diaries and letters. While recounting a discussion with a fellow married doctor, Adye-Curran wrote 'we chatted about many things, married life included and he agrees with me that it is the only way to live'.[86]

Twenty-six per cent of the contingent of married Irish doctors who enlisted in the British Army medical services during the First World War entered during the final two years of conflict as the RAMC's need for doctors increased following the Battle of the Somme, the Allied offensives on the Salonika Front and German attacks on hospital ships.[87] In March 1917, for instance, the IMWC commissioned Denis

O'Donoghue, a retired County Kerry doctor who was married, into the RAMC.[88] O'Donoghue's enlistment typifies the IMWC's recruitment procedures during the latter stages of the war and demonstrates that while the committee sought to commission an ideal candidate who was young and single, they were prepared to waive both requirements when the RAMC's need for medical manpower increased. The RAMC's requirements superseded any desire to adhere to a specific social profile.

## RELIGION AND EDUCATION

Recruitment committees also sought to use the religious affiliations of Irish men to encourage them into the British Army. In the opening months of the war, Ireland's newspapers, including the *Cork Free Press, Westmeath Examiner* and *The Newtownards Chronicle*, drew comparisons between the Catholic identities of Belgium and Ireland in the articles detailing the atrocities committed by the Germans against Belgium.[89] Recruiters utilised these stories in their literature to elicit a response from Ireland's Catholic population.[90] It is unclear whether any feelings of religious kinship with the Belgians encouraged Ireland's Catholic doctors to enlist. Yet it is evident that a significant number of Irish Catholic doctors joined the RAMC and other associated medical units of the British Army. Forty-five per cent of Irish doctors who participated in the British Army during the First World War and whose religious affiliation could be determined were Catholic (Fig. 3.3).

Irish Protestant doctors outnumbered their Catholic colleagues during the conflict but the rise in the number of Irish Catholic doctors in the British Army medical services was notable. In their study of British and Irish doctors who enlisted in the British Army between 1790 and 1850, Ackroyd et al., indicated that the majority of military medical officers during this period were Protestant, which reflected the religious loyalties of British society. However, they also estimated that nineteen per cent of recruits whose religious allegiance could be identified were Catholic and of those, almost all were Irish. Approximately one-third of Irish medical officers who enlisted in the British Army from 1790 to 1850 were Catholic.[91] It is important to acknowledge a significant caveat regarding the figures recorded in the nineteenth century, which were most likely conservative estimates at best. As Ackroyd et al., have argued, it was likely that some recruits lied about their religious affiliation during the enlistment process. King George III was reluctant to employ

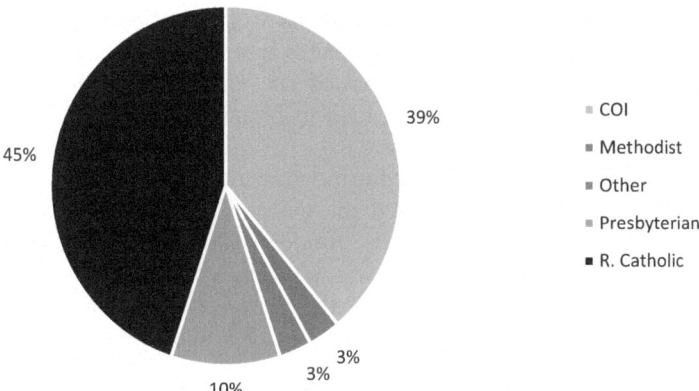

Fig. 3.3 Religious affiliation of Irish doctors who participated in the First World War (*Source* Database of Irish medical officers in British forces who served in the First World War—based on a sample of 800 doctors)

Catholics in the armed forces and it was possible that some of Ireland's medical men seeking a commission in the Army Medical Services felt obliged to change their religion to acquire an enlistment.[92] Even considering this complexity, it is still reasonable to claim that the proportion of Irish Catholic doctors in the British Army medical services increased during the First World War era. The need for medical manpower during the conflict eclipsed any religious prejudice that may have previously influenced the recruitment process.

The rise in the number of Irish Catholic middle-class men who received a medical education in Ireland was instrumental in their increased involvement in the British Army medical services. From the middle of the nineteenth century, there were significant changes to the availability and structure of medical education in Ireland. Introduced in 1845, the Queen's Colleges (Ireland) Act established three colleges in Belfast, Cork and Galway to provide non-denominational education in Ireland and these institutions included medical schools. The hierarchy of the Roman Catholic Church strongly opposed these 'godless colleges' and, in response, founded the Catholic University of Ireland in Dublin which opened in 1854.[93] Its medical school in Cecilia Street opened in 1855. The Catholic University did not have a charter and thus could not award degrees. Instead, medical students who were educated there often subsequently took the licences of the Royal College of Surgeons and the King and Queen's College of Physicians. Licences allowed students to practice medicine after they had passed the examinations but degrees, that took longer to achieve, were held in higher esteem by the medical profession.[94]

Further changes to higher education occurred in 1879 when the University Education Act founded the examining and degree-awarding Royal University of Ireland (RUI). Students could choose their place of education and the RUI then awarded degrees to those who passed its annual examinations. Soon after, the Catholic University was reorganised as University College, Dublin and its medical students began to take the examinations of the RUI.[95] In 1908, the RUI was dissolved under the terms of the Irish Universities Act and replaced by two separate examining institutions—the National University of Ireland (three constituent colleges: University College Cork, University College Dublin and University College Galway) and Queen's University Belfast (QUB). These universities were non-denominational. The National University was designed as a secular university that was acceptable to Catholics due to legal protection against interreference in religious beliefs and the presence of Catholics among the staff.[96] Due to the changes in higher education in Ireland, the number of Catholic medical graduates emerging from its universities increased. University College Dublin's medical school soon became the largest in Ireland.[97] The rise in the number of Catholic medical graduates in search of work thus ensured their increased involvement in the British Army medical services during the First World War.

The educational background of all Irish medical recruits, including Catholics, Protestants and those of other religious beliefs, was varied. As demonstrated in Fig. 3.4, many Irish doctors who enlisted in the British Army medical services graduated from TCD. This is perhaps unsurprising given TCD's successful medical school, Officer Training Corps and long-standing tradition of its graduates enlisting in the British Army and Colonial Services. More than 3000 staff, students and alumni of TCD joined the British Army and approximately one-third of those enlisted in the RAMC.[98] While the vast majority of the sample of Irish doctors received their medical education in Ireland, Britain, with its many medical courses and institutions, was also a popular option for Irish students. Dupree and Crowther have shown that Irish medical students enrolled in British universities throughout the nineteenth century.[99] This continued

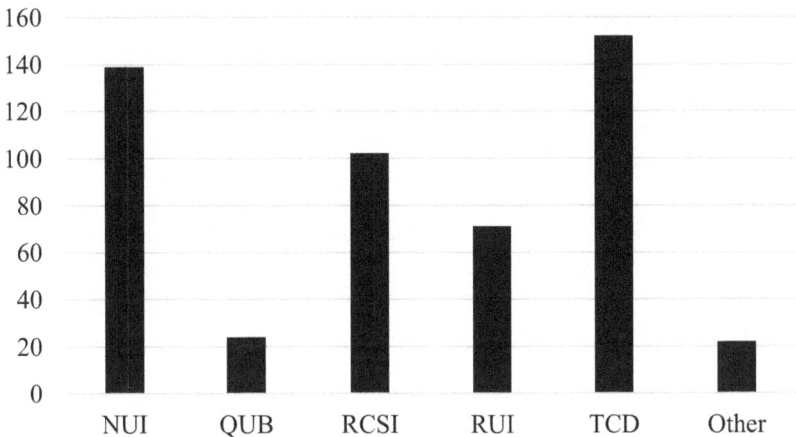

**Fig. 3.4** Educational background of Irish doctors who participated in the First World War (*Source* Database of Irish medical officers in British forces who served in the First World War—based on a sample of 500 doctors)

in the years immediately before the war. Figure 3.4 indicates that approximately five per cent of Irish doctors, who subsequently served in the British Army medical services during the First World War, were educated outside of Ireland's large medical schools and among this cohort were those who were educated in Britain. While this appears to be a rather low percentage, it is important to outline the complexities that surround this figure. The database of Irish doctors sampled in this study emerged primarily from an analysis of sources chiefly concerned with Irish medical personnel who graduated from Irish universities or had careers in Ireland.[100] As Kelly has demonstrated in her study of Irish medical students training at the University of Glasgow, those who were educated at universities abroad rarely returned home.[101] Therefore, there were additional Irish doctors educated in universities abroad who did not have careers in Ireland and subsequently enlisted in the British Army medical services who are not accounted for in the statistics listed here.

Both religious affiliation and educational background influenced Irish doctors' wartime experiences. Religion was a prominent feature of daily life on the battlefield for several of Ireland's medical personnel.[102] Stafford Adye-Curran noted in his wartime diary that 'without religion, life is useless'.[103] As part of his daily routine, Adye-Curran met with the local chaplain, visited nearby chapels and attended mass. As he moved from town to town, he made it a priority to locate the nearest church as quickly as possible; 'arrived in Belgium, went into the Cathedral, a lovely place, and said some prayers'.[104] He was displeased if either chaplain or the mass did not reach his high expectations—'I got up and went to mass. It is very difficult to be attentive as most of the people sing out of tune'.[105] Similarly, J. P. Lynch noted that he was able to go to mass every Sunday while in Torgan, France and that 'the French priest had arranged a nice little chapel in a loft over one of the barracks, we had an altar and a harmonium there and it was great thing for us to be able to go there'.[106]

A doctors' educational background and training also affected their wartime experiences. The RAMC educated its recruits to prepare them for war. Career army medics who had enlisted prior to August 1914 had their university medical education supplemented by courses of instruction in the RAMC's college where well-established army medics taught courses in sanitation, hygiene and casualty disposal.[107] The RAMC educated doctors who enlisted during the war at the medical training centres established by military authorities throughout Britain and Ireland. In Ireland, RAMC staff at two centres established in Newry City and County Tipperary trained the personnel of the FAs of the 10th and 16th Irish Divisions.[108] In 1916, following the mobilisation of both of these divisions, the RAMC expanded the objectives of the training centres to include the training of any reinforcement volunteers who came forward and personnel for CCS. By providing military training, both centres prepared Irish doctors', who had little to no experience of working in conflict, for service in the First World War.

Several doctors who enlisted also had previously received some military training at university. Surgeon General Russell, a member of the RAMC, informed the principal of Glasgow University that 'it has been clearly shown that men who have previous military training are of infinitely greater value as officers of the RAMC than those who have had no military experience'.[109] In 1908, the War Office, in association with TCD, formed the Dublin University Officer Training Corps, placed under the control of Major Tate. Similar to the army itself, the Training Corps was divided into several sections—infantry unit, army service corps, royal engineers and RAMC. In her study of TCD and the First World War, Laura Dooney likened the training corps to an athletics club but 'with added panoply of guns and uniforms'.[110] The corps was very popular among TCD's students—approximately half the student population actively participated.[111]

In 1909, the RCSI established its own Officer Training Corps at the request of its students. Similar to the corps at TCD, the RCSI contingent practiced military drills and the *Irish Times* reported that pedestrians in Nassau Street watched with interest the 'large musters' of men in uniform which often took place in the area.[112] For a training corps to be of any benefit to its members, it was important for it to have experienced members providing necessary instruction. At the RCSI, Professor Auckland Geddes, member of staff and veteran of British Army medical services' campaigns in South Africa, provided training to students in the corps. Geddes advised on military drills, presented lectures and brought recruits on camp training.[113] The importance of these training corps to the War Office and RAMC was twofold: firstly, it allowed RAMC hierarchy to gauge the response of Irish medical personnel to the prospect of enlisting in the British Army medical services; secondly, by adding basic military training to the subjects already taught by the medical faculties, the Officer Training Corps somewhat prepared Ireland's medical students for the complex wartime arrangements implemented by the British Army medical services during the First World War.

## THE EXPERIENCES OF IRISH MEDICAL PERSONNEL IN THE FIRST WORLD WAR

Irish doctors' experience of the First World War began on 30 July 1914, when RAMC hierarchy instructed the MOs already enlisted in the corps to begin mobilising. Harrison, in his analysis of the RAMC's First World War medical infrastructure, argued that Britain's wartime medical arrangements resembled a 'medical machine'.[114] Certainly, the scale and detail of the administrative and organisational work undertaken by the British Army medical services during the First World War was unprecedented. The maintenance of effective techniques and processes of casualty evacuation from the frontlines back to hospitals and wards in Britain and Ireland required extensive planning and precision.

Figure 3.5 illustrates an evacuation chain on a Western Front battlefield. Stretcher-bearers collected injured soldiers from combat zones and carried them to the nearest Regimental Aid Post—a zone occupied by RAMC MOs, often located in shell craters or structural ruins—before transporting the wounded to Advanced Dressing Stations. Here, injured

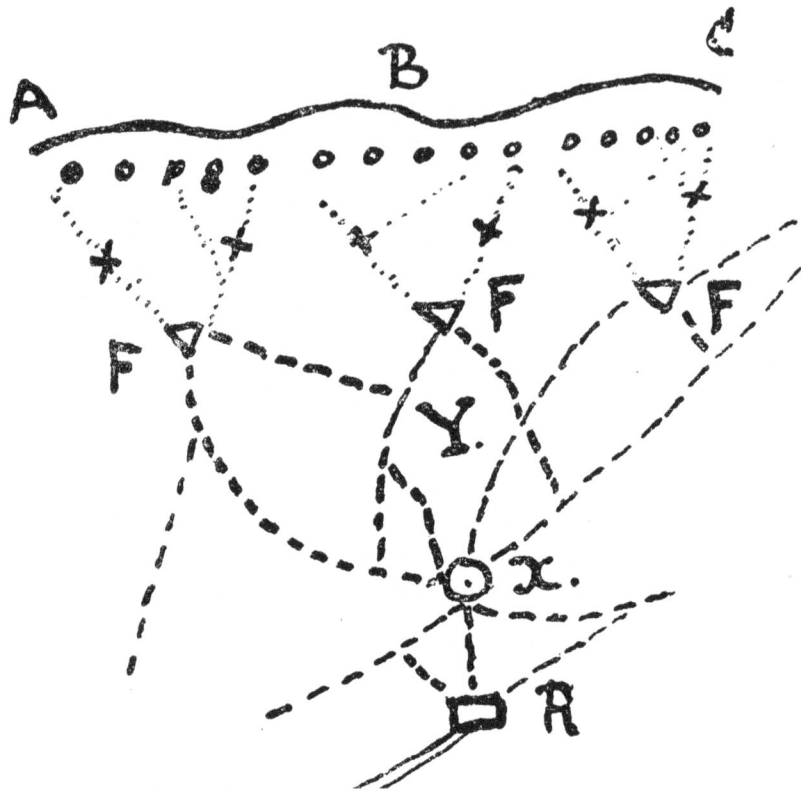

A, B, C, Portion of a battle line.  o o o, Aid posts of battalions in action.  × × ×, Advanced dressing stations  F F F, Field ambulance tent or head quarter sections.  x, Casualty clearing station. R, Railhead.  =, Line of communication with base.  ......, Paths available for bearer parties.  – – – –, Roads.

**Fig. 3.5** Portion of a battle line, outlining casualty clearing stations diagram showing the position of casualty clearing stations (*Source*: *British Medical Journal*, December 1915. *Credit* Wellcome Collection. CC BY)

soldiers had their wounds dressed and were then transported by FA—horse-drawn carriages or motor vehicles—to a CCS. RAMC personnel in the CCS dealt with injuries requiring immediate treatment and conducted numerous surgical procedures. Ambulance cars and trains then transported the wounded fit for transportation to nearby hospitals established by the RAMC or voluntary groups, such as the Red Cross. MOs also identified soldiers requiring treatment in hospitals on the homefront and recommended these men be moved, by hospital ship, back to domestic hospitals in Britain and Ireland.[115] Significant numbers of medical personnel occupied roles at each stage of the casualty clearing process and Irish doctors and nurses were among them since the outbreak of war.

Following mobilisation instructions, MOs already enlisted in the corps travelled to their local barracks for a medical examination. J. P. Lynch recalled travelling to his local Canterbury barracks and examining his colleagues after he had been passed fit. Lynch recounts a tale of having to go 'round the town to hunt up doctors to help in the examination'.[116] Once a recruit passed their medical examination, they were deployed from their nearest depot. Some of the first RAMC deployments travelled directly from Dublin to France. On 18 August 1914, No. 1 Stationary Hospital, No. 1 General Hospital and three FA Divisions (numbers 13, 14 and 15) departed Dublin for Le Havre. On the same date, two other FAs (16 and 17) departed from Cork for Saint-Nazaire in western France.[117] Within four weeks of the War Office's mobilisation orders, many of Ireland's RAMC doctors had been transported to France along with ambulance wagons, horses and water carts. The doctors' initial reactions to the wartime conditions of work varied depending on the jobs assigned to them.

Irish medical personnel fulfilled several different roles in the RAMC's chain of evacuation. Their wartime experiences varied significantly depending on their role, location and the battles occurring in their locality. Shortly after the outbreak of war, the RAMC appointed Stafford Adye-Curran as Regimental Medical Officer (RMO) to the 17th Lancers who arrived in France in late November. An RMO provided medical care to their assigned unit by positioning themselves in the aid posts nearest the battle-lines. They travelled with their unit on all assignments. Adye-Curran complained that constant travelling and waiting for orders was a source of much frustration—'I believe tomorrow we will arrive at Boulogne. Actually, to where I am going I don't know. It may seem somewhat interesting to be on a train and not know where you are going but it's dull really'.[118]

An RMO, based near the frontline, could find himself deeply involved in the casualty clearing process on the battlefield, particularly if they acted as a regiment's stretcher-bearer, which many did in the early months of the war.[119] Whitehead has argued that doctors had a problem with RMO work because of its sporadic nature—quiet at one moment and overworked the next.[120] The wartime experiences of Irish RMOs certainly confirmed that this was the case. In November 1914, Richard Hingston, who enlisted in the IMS, served as a RMO in a small town close to Bombay. Hingston was no stranger to conflict having served with the IMS for a number of years prior to war. On 10 November 1914, however, he noted that

> I have been present at spectacles which for the first time, have given me a timely impression of the real horrors of war. All day long on the 4<sup>th</sup> we could see the glint of bayonets and hear the rattle of the machine guns and rifle fire ... at dusk an urgent message came demanding every medical officer that could possibly be spared ... On our arrival at the hospital, chaos and confusion reigned supreme. Wounded, dying and dead strewed the ground in all directions ... every shed was packed to overflowing with the wounded; all the spare ground, both inside and behind the house was profusely littered with them. Hundreds lay all around. This was nothing to those that were scattered through the jungle. No beds, no blankets, no water, no food. The wounded arrived in so fast that there was scarcely time to apply the simplest dressings; no operation but the most urgent amputations could be performed and these only under the most unfavourable circumstances ... the wounded were groaning and crying, the place was red with blood.[121]

In contrast, Adye-Curran's time as an RMO was characterised by long periods of inactivity. Despite being based near the frontlines, he often found himself with little to do:

> we are now well up the firing line and one hears the rattle of rifles and occasional shells bursting ... I had a look at the German trenches through field glasses. They could be seen quite distinctly and their observation post, which was in a church tower, we were a couple of hundred yards from them ... no orders came in for me.[122]

Adye-Curran spent his time in his living quarters rather than on the battlefield and the constant change of living arrangements annoyed him: 'I asked the lady of the brewery if she could let me have a room ... five francs a month of course. It is an utter shame these French people seem to think we are here for amusement. Well I wish I had never seen their rotten country'.[123] Hingston and Adye-Curran's time as RMOs demonstrate the varied wartime experiences of doctors occupying similar roles.

Adye-Curran's 'lack of action' was not an isolated case as doctors often complained about the RAMC's misuse of medical manpower on the Western Front in the early years of the war. In October 1915, at a meeting between the CMWC and Sir Alfred Keogh, the committee presented Keogh with complaints from a British medical man at the front who criticised the RAMC for their failure to fully utilise doctors correctly; the recruit argued that there was often little for him to do.[124] Doctors were eager to utilise their professional skill while at war; this was often borne out in their diaries and letters. On 15 August 1915, the RAMC appointed Eugene Ryan to take over from Lieutenant Colonel John David Ferguson RAMC as Commanding Officer of No. 18 CCS located at Lapugnoy, France. He noted in a letter sent to his wife that 'I am glad I am going as I will have much more interesting work'.[125]

Inactivity in war caused mental strain for a number of doctors. Adye-Curran's idleness during the early months of the conflict initiated an apparent bout of depression. Early parts of his wartime diary are characterised by gloomy statements—'I again went to report myself but there was no orders and I returned to the hotel feeling very depressed and completely fed up with life in general'[126]; 'did not hear any firing today. I saw a few aeroplanes. Hope for a better tomorrow'.[127] Joanna Bourke, among others, has investigated shell-shock in the First World War.[128] She has argued that most men who suffered from the condition in war never killed anyone and that the passivity of wartime experiences was unbearable for some recruits.[129] Lieutenant Colonel Charles Burtchaell had made similar claims in a 1920 address to the Royal Academy of Medicine in Ireland, insisting that soldiers in the combat forces regularly broke down while out of the firing line.[130] An extension of these arguments are applicable to medical personnel. This is not to say that doctors harboured any deep desire or need to kill, rather, many needed to work to stave off the mental distress that appears to have characterised inactivity. Richard Hingston, who had been in the thick of the action during the early months of war, acknowledged that he suffered from a deep depression as a consequence of inactivity after his reassignment to Basra:

> what a year of sorrow and destruction to the world; and for myself what a year of worthlessness and waste! Looking back on the past two years, solely from a personal and selfish standpoint, I find them to be years completely thrown away ... The very writing of a journal is a burden; memory is failing, very little enthusiasm for anything remains. These are the

early symptoms of that mental depression that follows too long a residence in this monotonous climate and which is often characterised as 'Basra Head'.[131]

Of course, not all Irish doctors' wartime experiences were characterised by depression and idleness. Several regularly recorded being overworked, including those dispersed throughout various FA divisions. When active, an FA was one of the busiest medical units involved in the war. Thomas Gordon, in his address to the students union of the RCSI, recounted a tale about a friend who was in charge of an FA in Ypres. The friend had informed him how in one day they had dressed 300 men to send off as quickly as possible to the hospital train, in order to make room for more. Gordon asserted that 'it's not surgery, under these conditions—it is packing'.[132] Those in command of an FA required administrative skill to overcome the various difficulties involved. These included the shortage of transport, equipment failure, navigation troubles and unsuitable roads and routes. The RAMC and the medical profession debated whether university-educated doctors were suited to this role given the substantial administrative work.[133] Yet, the RAMC hierarchy insisted that it was essential to have men with medical qualifications and expertise in control.

Irish doctors commanded FA divisions throughout the war. On 22 August 1914, for instance, Captain J. P. Lynch commanded the 4th FA, which travelled to the town of La Longueville in northern France. Lynch was responsible for the efficient dispersal of manpower and ambulances within his unit and was under severe pressure due to heavy fighting in the town:

> on arriving we opened up for the reception of the sick and had quite a busy afternoon ... a few of the cases were temporarily unfit, and I intended to send them to the base on the first opportunity ... but there was no empty supply lorries in the evening so they remained over.[134]

An ambulance division was regularly on the move. On 26 August 1914, a brigade major ordered Lynch to lead his ambulance units to Landrecy, a town near Longneville, to evacuate the wounded. Lynch noted 'there are 160 killed and wounded ... collect and evacuate the wounded and bury the dead ... the whole Field Ambulance must go back'.[135]

The unpredictable nature of FA work appealed to some Irish doctors. In 1914, Henry Moore, a County Louth doctor and RCSI graduate, after volunteering for service, entered an FA Division based in France. During the course of the war, Moore turned down several promotions because they would have taken him away from the FA and 'front-line work'.[136] On 21 April 1915, the RAMC reassigned Stafford Adye-Curran to an FA and his mood noticeably changed: 'got charge of the motor ambulance cars (just what I wanted) ... I like this class of work'.[137] In contrast to his days spent as an RMO, his assignment in the FA division brought a new daily routine and a completely new set of responsibilities. His excitement at his new role was clear:

> I am to go up tomorrow and take charge of the Lucknow [Field Ambulance unit]. I have ten officers under me. I am writing this in my little room and needless to say I feel very excited as it is a big undertaking and I feel anxious that all will go well ... I feel that there is a tide in the affairs of man so I must take it at the flood or be left. The 1st of June will be a big day in my life.[138]

Within a day of taking charge, RAMC hierarchy passed down 'unexpected orders to move [his division] at once'.[139] His diary entries, which were almost daily during his time as an RMO, reduced after his reassignment: 'have not had a moment to write'.[140] His experiences in charge of the FA division also brought him in close contact with the frontlines as his unit retrieved men from battle-torn regions. His appointment coincided with the beginning of the Second Battle of Ypres and on his first day in command, he travelled to the region:

> It is a most extraordinary sight, [the area] was still burning. We did not stop too long as the shells were beginning to pop around and we cleared out ... it would be impossible to describe all the sights – trenches, barbed wire, armoured cars patrolling the roads on the lookout for aeroplanes, troops, batteries. The roads were all cut up with shell holes.[141]

In several cases, an FA fulfilled dual roles in the process of evacuation. Adye-Curran's unit, for example, also established an Advanced Dressing Station during their time in Ypres. An Advanced Dressing Station primarily acted as a treatment centre for the wounded before they were transported on to more established base hospitals. During

bombardments, those working in dressing stations often delayed transporting casualties, as it was too dangerous to move men to the next stage
of the process.[142] On 7 June 1915, Adye-Curran established a station in
a school; he acknowledged that 'it makes a good dressing station so long
as they don't drop any shells onto it. We have made everything fairly nice
and are ready to take in a large number of patients'.[143] A dressing station
was often one of the most hectic stops on the evacuation line, particularly during large battles:

> very busy all afternoon. The King's Dragoon Guards had been so badly
> shelled that they had to come back. I believe they have about 60 casual-
> ties, 2 officers killed, 2 wounded and several sergeants killed … Got in two
> officers who had been hit by shell near Ypres. One was killed, the other in
> an awful state, don't expect he will live. Both legs injured and half thigh
> blown away – we have been working hard all day … have not had clothes
> off for three days.[144]

An FA transferred wounded soldiers requiring additional treatment
to base hospitals located on the lines of evacuation. Richard Hingston
described his experience working in an IMS hospital based in Tanga, a
military post in East Africa:

> the wounded arrived in so fast that there was scarcely time to apply the
> simplest dressings; no operation but the most urgent amputations could
> be performed and these only under the most unfavourable circumstances.
> The iron sheds were like shambles … all of us were busy; far into the
> night we were dressing wounds, amputating limbs, injecting, doing all
> that was humanly possible for the comfort of the wounded. This little
> makeshift hospital and small staff could scarcely cope with such a burst of
> wounded.[145]

To support the work of the doctors along the lines of evacuation,
groups of nurses assisted with the medical care of the sick and wounded.
Irish women enlisted in large numbers into the various nursing corps.
As explained, it is difficult to detail an exact number of Irish military
nurses and VADs who participated in the war, however, Clear has suggested that approximately 4500 Irish nurses served abroad.[146] Ireland's
nurses provided medical care to soldiers from the outbreak of conflict.
In August 1914, a ship carrying a full contingent of nurses sailed from
Dublin for the war.[147] They joined with other national groups of trained

military nurses who enlisted from elsewhere including Australia, Canada, New Zealand and South Africa, and served in several locations such as France, Malta, Salonika and Gallipoli.[148]

Both professional and VAD Irish nurses participated in the conflict. Janet Watson has argued that the approach to treatment of an experienced professional nurse who had already worked in various general and military hospitals differed from that of an inexperienced volunteer.[149] According to her memoir, Catherine Black from County Donegal was a trained nurse who enlisted with the British Army nursing service to participate in the First World War. She decided to become a nurse at a young age and when she reached her late teens, travelled to a hospital in a large sea-side town on the south coast of England to become a probationer. She worked in the London Hospital when the war began. Black claimed that 'like most people I thought it would be all over by Christmas'.[150] She signed up for the QAIMNS and was initially assigned to the Cambridge Hospital at Aldershot where she helped treat soldiers suffering from facial wounds which she noted were 'the saddest injuries' she had to deal with during the war. She recalled in her memoir that these injuries were even sadder than those she witnessed in the CCS as there 'death was swifter and more merciful, and it is not so hard to see a man die as to break the news to him that he will be blind and dumb for the rest of his life'.[151] In autumn 1916, Black was assigned to No. 7 General Hospital, an old converted monastery in St. Omer in northern France. Black was in charge of a ward for shell-shocked officers.[152]

Marie Martin was twenty-three when she applied and was called up to serve with the VADs in Malta.[153] In 1916, Albert MacKinnon, a British clergyman in the Church of England, labelled Malta with the moniker 'nurse of the Mediterranean' due to the high concentration of medical facilities located there during the war.[154] Medical services established twenty-seven hospitals and camps there. Martin travelled on the hospital ship *Oxfordshire* and arrived in Malta on 22 October 1915. The Red Cross assigned her to a converted barracks of approximately 840 beds on a peninsula overlooking St. George's Bay on the northern shore of the island a few miles from Valetta. She was the only Irish VAD in her contingent.[155]

Black and Martin's wartime experiences differed in many respects, not only because they were both located in different regions but because Black was a trained nurse and Martin a VAD. Both women approached their duties in a noticeably different manner. Hallett and Fell have suggested that professional nurses were trained to maintain a safe emotional distance between themselves and their patients. While VADs, without such training and experience, were more likely to engage with their patients in a friendly manner.[156] Black's and Martin's recorded wartime experiences support this thesis. Black noted upon her arrival in St. Omer that at first sight most of her patients appeared to have little or nothing the matter with them. They were just the average, healthy, young men. However, at night, she recalls, that

> the cheerful ward became a place of torment, with the occupant of every bed tossing a turning and moaning in a hell of memories let loose. And there was so little one could do to help them. Our chief difficulty was that we had always to work more or less in the dark, for no two shell-shock cases were ever the same, and one man would respond favourably to treatment that would be disastrous for another.[157]

To treat those suffering from shell-shock, Black and her fellow doctors and nurses 'gave sufferers opiates for a week or ten days to encourage the men to rest'.[158] The care following the prescription of opiates 'demanded endless patience' as each case had to be dealt with on an individual basis and there was little in the way of treatment patterns.[159] Black's recollection of the events and her role in the process suggest that she maintained an emotional distance from the patient and focused solely on carrying out her role as a nurse. Martin, on the other hand, spent a lot of her time engaging with the patients. She recalled that she spent her time off work in Malta writing letters for ill patients and listening to their stories of the harsh conditions they had faced in battle.[160]

Similar to the doctors, nurses—professional and VADs—struggled to deal with the workload in a busy CCS. On 28 October 1915, in a letter to her mother, Martin stated that 'the work is really hard, but of course it is what we came out for'.[161] Nurses, like others in the CCS, were in danger from enemy fire. After a year in St. Omer, Black was moved to Poperinghe, in West Flanders, where she was needed to cover for eight nurses who had been injured, one fatally, after a bomb was dropped on a CCS.[162] On Black's first morning in Poperinghe, she had to work knee-deep in water following a heavy downpour of rain during the previous night that had flooded the facility. She maintained that

> I know that they (Casualty Clearing Stations) changed us. You could not go through the things we went through, see the things we saw, and remain

the same. You went into it young and light-hearted. You came out older than any span of years could make you. But at the time you did not reflect on it much, or on anything else...you were an experienced nurse; you had been chosen to serve at a CCS because of that, and you were supposed to be used to grim sights and sounds and smells. But even so, there was so much that no nursing experience in the world could have prepared you for.[163]

Both Black and Martin's work was intense at certain points throughout the war and Black's recollection of her time in the CCS raises questions as to whether experiences on the casualty evacuation line influenced the attitudes of Irish medical personnel—nurses and doctors—towards the war.

Certainly, medical personnel were affected by what they observed at war. Witnessing first-hand the illnesses of, and injuries to, soldiers, and the death of colleagues often increased patriotism and belief in the British war effort. As badly wounded men returned to medical tents, FA divisions and hospitals, hostility towards Germans emerged among Irish medical personnel who staffed these units.[164] Adye-Curran, for example, displayed utter contempt for the Germans: 'the Germans have played so many low down games that he only deserves to be shot like a dog as soon as he is found'.[165]

Some German officers, aware of the Irish campaign for self-government, attempted to stir up divisions between British and Irish troops to undermine this anti-German sentiment among the Irish and to cause division in the British Army. This was evident on 26 August 1914, when a group of German infantry seized Lynch and his FA division in the town of Landrecies, France. Kept as prisoners of war (POW) for over a year, they were transported to POW camps and treated harshly on route: 'we met some German artillery on the march ... I hope they will be exterminated in the war because these men were brutes ... [they] cursed at us, lashed at us with their long whips ... and cursed me in English and in German'.[166] Shortly after arriving at a POW camp in Burg bei Magdeburg, Germany, a commanding officer of the camp ordered Lynch and all Irish Catholics to fall out of line. Officers marched these men to a room isolated from British POWs. Members from other Irish regiments had been placed in this room before the group arrived. The Commandant of Burg then held a court enquiry into whether the Royal Munster Fusiliers, an Irish regiment of the British Army, had attacked the King's Own Scottish Borderers (KOSB), a British regiment, in retaliation for an attack by the KOSBs on a mob in Dublin. Lynch, the Munsters and all other Irish POWs refuted the allegations as untrue. However according to Lynch, 'it was too good a story from a German point of view – the KOSBs had been so easily wiped out by the Munsters, who in their turn were smashed up by the irresistible German army'.[167] Following their refusal to corroborate the story, the camp authorities moved Irish POWs to stables and gun sheds 'not fit for human habitation' for the remainder of their stay.[168]

## 1916 RISING

Following the 1916 Easter Rising, Irish recruits came under increasing scrutiny from key figures within the British Army. On 2 July 1916, Sir Henry Rawlinson, British Commander of 4th Army, criticised the Irish rebels for attempting to capitalise on the British government's weakness during the middle of the war, 'when all the buggers should be devoted to winning it'. He argued that among Irishmen, 'there are very few who [are loyal]. Down in the warren of their loins is a dislike ... this appeared to have somewhat died down. But it was there all the time and always will be there'.[169] Yet the Rising had little effect on the wartime experiences of Irish doctors serving in the British Army. Myles Dungan has argued that the details of the Easter Rising took considerable time to filter through to the nationalist 16th division and there was little in the way of demonstrations or desertions.[170] Similarly, Jane Leonard interviewed a number of Irish First World War veterans from the other divisions and found that the majority had 'little or no recollection of exactly when they heard about the Rising'.[171] The same was true in the army medical services. The Rising had the potential to cause division among British and Irish doctors, and indeed unionist and nationalist Irish doctors, in the army medical services. Yet Irish wartime doctors were more concerned with their wartime duties and offered little in the way of opinion on the Rising, despite being aware of it. On 17 May 1916, Richard Hingston, based in the city of Nasiriyah in the Ottoman Empire, recorded in his diary that 'today's mail brought us the report of the fall of Kut and the Irish rebellion', yet he offered no judgement on the matter.[172] Instead, his diary entries focus on the battles and events immediately surrounding him including the Battle of Sahilan and casualty evacuations to Basra.

Relations between Irish and British doctors within the army remained cordial, even after the outbreak of the Rising. Evidence shows that doctors in the British Army medical services sometimes displayed contempt for medical personnel from other nations. For example, Tyquin has argued that tensions between Australian and British doctors developed because of a lack of communication between the two groups coupled with the fact that the Australian Army Medical Corps was forced to act as a subservient unit to the RAMC.[173] Similarly, Peter Rees has contended that Anzac nurses had a difficult relationship with English officers and surgeons.[174] However, Irish doctors had no such problems and there were several reasons for this: firstly, unlike their Australian counterparts, Irish doctors did not form their own medical corps. Instead, the RAMC absorbed Irish medical men into their unit and therefore Irish doctors had equal status with their British colleagues. They were assigned the same duties, afforded the same benefits and had the same opportunities of receiving the same honours and awards as British wartime doctors.[175] On 11 September 1916, the War Office awarded Hingston the Military Cross for bravery in the field. He was elated at the news, claiming that 'it is gratifying to know that one can face the music with credit and that one is labelled against an accusation of timidity ... Everyone treats you with more respect; is more inclined to be obliging'.[176] For the most part, parity of treatment between British and Irish medical men prevented problems arising between the two groups.

Secondly, and perhaps most importantly, for the thirty-five per cent of Irish doctors who were career army medics prior to the outbreak of the First World War, their involvement in the British Army medical services was unexceptional. Bonds between these doctors from every province in Ireland and their British colleagues had formed over the years. During mobilisation, Lynch noted that he was 'back at the old hospital. Very glad to see all my old friends again'.[177] Likewise, Adye-Curran recounted several stories of running into old colleagues, 'I met Colonel Thomas Wade, Lancashire Fusiliers. He recognised me at once. We were together in Trinidad'.[178] On 26 July 1916, Hingston recalled how he met a member of his extended family for the first time:

> was sent to medical reinforcement camp [in Basra] to await orders. There I met a Captain Hingston, RAMC, one of the English members of the family. He was almost as ignorant as myself of the shoots and branches of the family tree ... he had for years been hoping to find a member of the Irish Hingstons. How strange that we should meet on the fringe of the Mesopotamia desert.[179]

In many ways, it was essential for Irish doctors to maintain good relationships with all men in their unit, regardless of nationality or political background. Cooperation among members of the British Army medical services was required to overcome the difficulties presented by the dangerous wartime environment. On 5 June 1915, Adye-Curran based in Ypres, recalled how on a journey with another FA division, he pleaded for his fellow commanding officer to alter their route:

> I refused to go any further until I was certain [of the way] and looked at the map. Just as we stopped the car, a shell burst about 40 yards in front and fairly banged us all. As soon as I knew no one was hurt we hurriedly backed the cars. I told them that always the Germans dropped a couple of shells in the same place. I had only backed the cars when another dropped and burst over [where we had been]. I was jolly glad when we got home.[180]

Without cooperation between the two divisions, it was likely that both groups would have been shelled.

Adye-Curran's story also demonstrates the dangers Irish doctors experienced during the war. Thomas Gibbon was a captain in the RAMC and RMO for the KOSB regiment in France in the early weeks of the war. On 9 October, he wrote to his brother in Dublin to inform him that he had been wounded while administering treatment to the regiment:

> A few odd bullets kept dropping about in the field and after a time an odd horse or two was hit. I tried to see if we could get back a bit but we found that all the ground behind us was more or less being swept by machine gun fire so that there was not a chance of moving. It was shortly after this about 3.30 that I got hit myself. It was just like getting a very hard hit on the leg. It was not particularly pleasant as it was fairly close to my anterior tibial nerve. I could not make out where the bullet had come out and it was not till I had got my gaiter off that I discovered that the bullet was still in my leg.[181]

In total, approximately ten per cent of the sample of Irish doctors who served with the British Army medical services during the First World War died during the conflict.[182] The morality rate and the cause of deaths of doctors was attributable to the changing nature and location of warfare.

In 1914, Irish doctors were most likely to die due to bullet related injuries and subsequent infection. In the early months of the war, most Irish doctors served with the RAMC alongside the British Expeditionary Force and took part in intensive battles—Battle of the Frontiers (August 1914), Battle of Le Cateau (August 1914), Battle of the Marne (September 1914), and the Battle of Aisne (September 1914).[183] Illness, infection and disease, often stemming from inadequate surgical techniques, plagued the British Forces in France. British surgeons struggled to treat wounds that had become infected by the harmful microbes contained in French soil and many British troops died.[184] Medical personnel in the line of fire suffered from similar complications. Seventy-three per cent of Irish doctors who died in 1914 perished as a consequence of wounds. Charles Dalton, a lieutenant colonel in the RAMC from County Tipperary, died after he was seriously wounded by a shell and consequently developed gangrene.[185] William Gordon Cummings, who left his private practice in County Tyrone to participate in the war, was killed in action by a shell dropped in a crater in which he was attending to a wounded soldier.[186]

Disease and illness, including influenza, malaria, pneumonia and enteric fever, also caused a high proportion of deaths among Irish doctors. The diseases that caused deaths were usually prevalent in a doctor's assigned area. In 1915, dysentery was rife among troops during the Gallipoli campaign. 800 cases were evacuated from the area every day and enteric infection was rife.[187] Irish doctors serving in Gallipoli campaign shared in this suffering. In 1915, Bertram Letts, a County Down doctor, died of dysentery contracted during his time with the army in the Dardanelles.[188] Malaria was a significant concern for the RAMC in Malta throughout 1916.[189] In that year, fever caused the death of Reginald Holmes, an Irish RAMC captain who contracted the illness while serving in the region.[190] The number of deaths among Irish medical men and the wide-ranging causes exemplify the dangers faced by Ireland's RAMC doctors during the First World War.

## CONCLUSION

It has been posited here that Irish doctors enlisted in the British Army medical services for many of the same reasons as regular soldiers— economic motives and a belief in a just war—but that additional factors, which applied solely to medical men, also encouraged them to join up. Most notably, doctors enlisted because they believed that it was their duty to do so due to their professional skill and to ease suffering humanity. Self-mobilisation, which Horne has argued was evident in Britain, France and Germany, was central to motivating members of the Irish medical profession to enlist. Self-mobilisation among doctors and nurses continued largely because of the presence of the IMWC and peer pressure. At regular meetings of the medical profession, such as graduating ceremonies, societal or sporting events, doctors and nurses discussed the First World War and heralded and encouraged participation.

Given the findings of the analysis of social profile, it is argued that the social background of recruits provides further insight into the motivations behind the involvement of the medical men in the war. In an escalation of pre-war trends, analysed by Jones, many wartime recruits were young and newly qualified and thus sought to take advantage of the career opportunities offered by the RAMC in an overcrowded medical profession. The analysis of social profile has also identified continuities in the backgrounds of Irish doctors who enlisted in the British Army in the nineteenth century, detailed in the study by Ackroyd et al., and those who joined in the First World War. The most significant of these is that the sizeable recruitment of Protestant Irish medics into the forces, which had been evident in the nineteenth century, continued during the First World War. However, differences have also been identified, including the increase in the number of Catholic recruits. This chapter has thus argued that the rising number of Catholics receiving medical education, which occurred throughout the nineteenth and early twentieth century, was largely responsible for increasing the number of Irish Catholic doctors in the British Army during the First World War.

Moreover, this chapter has demonstrated that the wartime experiences of Irish MOs largely mirrored those of their British colleagues. Similar to British doctors, Irish medical involvement on the battlefields varied depending on assignment but there were often complaints of inactivity and frustration at an apparent lack of action.[191] It has also been shown that British and Irish doctors held equal standing within the RAMC. While Tyquin and Rees have found that Australian doctors and nurses had poor relations with their British colleagues, there is little evidence that Irish doctors experienced similar forms of discrimination, even after the 1916 Easter Rising.

# NOTES

1. Diaries of Stafford Adye-Curran, 10 April 1915 (NLI, MS 34,393).
2. Anon., 'Trinity College, Dublin and the war' in *British Medical Journal*, 2814, no. 2 (1914), p. 996.
3. Jones, 'Strike out boldly', pp. 55–74; Steven O'Connor, *Irish officers in the British forces, 1922–45* (Basingstoke: Palgrave Macmillan, 2014), pp. 83–107.
4. Jeffery, *Ireland and the Great War*, pp. 5–36; Fitzpatrick, 'The logic of collective sacrifice', pp. 1017–1030.
5. Fitzpatrick, 'The logic of collective sacrifice', pp. 1017–1030.
6. Jeffery, *Ireland and the Great War*, p. 10.
7. Marcus Ackroyd, Laurence Brockliss, Michael Moss, Kate Retford, and John Stevenson, *Advancing with the army: Medicine, the professions and social mobility in the British Isles, 1790–1850* (Oxford: Oxford University Press, 2006).
8. Whitehead, *Doctors in the Great War*, pp. 181–217; Harrison, *The medical war*, pp. 16–64.
9. See Harrison, *The medical war*, pp. 16–64.
10. Tyquin, *Little by little*, p. 130.
11. As examined by Whitehead in *Doctors in the Great War*, pp. 181–217.
12. Diaries of J. P. Lynch, 4 August 1914 (Wellcome Library [Hereafter WL], RAMC 453).
13. Jones, 'Strike out boldly', p. 71.
14. Digby, *Making a medical living*, p. 140. For more, see Irvine Loudon, 'Two thousand medical men in 1847' in *Bulletin of the Society for the Social History of Medicine*, 33 (1983), p. 4.
15. F. O. C. Meenan, *Cecilia Street: The Catholic University School of Medicine, 1855–1931* (Dublin: Gill and Macmillan, 1987), p. 4.
16. Charles Keetly, *The student's guide to the medical profession* (London: Macmillan, 1878) cited in Jones, 'Strike out boldly', p. 68.
17. Catherine Cox, 'The medical marketplace', p. 64.
18. Jones, 'Strike out boldly', p. 74; Also see *Report of the committee to inquire into the causes which tend to prevent sufficient eligible candidates from coming forward to the Army Medical Department* [C 2200], H.C. 1878–1879, XLIV, 1–55.
19. Jones, 'Strike out boldly', p. 72.
20. Whitehead, *Doctors in the Great War*, p. 47.
21. Digby, *Making a medical living*, p. 143.
22. *Southern Star*, 1 May 1915.
23. South Dublin Union Board of Guardians minute book, 5 February 1915 (NAI, MFGS 49/89).

24. House of Industry Hospitals minute book, 18 September 1914 (NAI, 2006/86).
25. House of Industry Hospitals minute book, 2 October 1914 (NAI, 2006/86).
26. *Limerick Leader*, 27 October 1915.
27. *Limerick Leader*, 27 October 1915.
28. *Limerick Leader*, 27 October 1915.
29. Fitzpatrick, 'The logic of collective sacrifice', p. 1021; Jeffery, *Ireland and the Great War*, p. 18.
30. David Fitzpatrick, 'The logic of collective sacrifice', p. 1030.
31. Anon., 'Conditions of leave to poor law medical officers joining the Royal Army Medical Corps' in *British Medical Journal*, 2874, no. 1 (1916), p. 181.
32. *Freeman's Journal*, 3 December 1915.
33. Phillip Orr, *The road to the Somme: Men of the Ulster Division tell their story* (Belfast: Blackstaff Press, 1987), p. 38.
34. Abraham, *Surgeon's journey*, p. 133.
35. *Freeman's Journal*, 1 April 1915.
36. *Irish Times*, 22 December 1916.
37. *Irish Times*, 22 December 1916.
38. *Southern Star*, 1 May 1915.
39. O'Connor, *Irish officers in the British forces*, p. 99.
40. Anon., 'Deputy Surgeon-General William Cherry, RAMC' in *British Medical Journal*, 2964, no. 2 (1917), p. 541.
41. Stafford Adye-Curran (RCPI, Kirkpatrick Index, TPCK/5/3).
42. Jeffery, *Ireland and the Great War*, p. 10.
43. Anon., 'Immediate need of doctors for the army' in *British Medical Journal*, 3015, no. 2 (1918), p. 417.
44. Postcards from Doran of Dublin to his family in Ireland while serving with the Royal Army Medical Corps (hereafter RAMC) in France (NLI, MS 24,581).
45. Diaries of Stafford Adye-Curran, 25 June 1915 (NLI, MS 34,393).
46. Thomas E. Gordon, 'The Great European War' in *Dublin Journal of Medical Science*, cxxxix (1915), p. 28.
47. *Freeman's Journal*, 1 April 1915.
48. John Horne, 'Mobilizing for Total War' in John Horne (ed.), *State, society and mobilization in Europe during the First World War* (Cambridge: Cambridge University Press, 1997), p. 5.
49. *Freeman's Journal*, 1 April 1915.
50. Anon., 'Ulster medical society' in *British Medical Journal*, 2840, no. 1 (1915), p. 988.
51. *Irish Times*, 2 November 1916.

52. Anon., 'Base Hospitals in Egypt' in *British Medical Journal*, 2916, no. 2 (1916), p. 702.
53. Anon., 'Ireland' in *British Medical Journal*, 2916, no. 2 (1916), p. 702.
54. Colin Cousins, *Armagh and the Great War* (Dublin: The History Press Ireland, 2011), p. 63.
55. Fitzpatrick, 'The logic of collective sacrifice', p. 1030.
56. Anthony Quinn, *Wigs and guns: Irish barristers in the Great War* (Dublin: Four Courts Press, 2006), p. 28.
57. Quinn, *Wigs and guns*, p. 28.
58. Book of newspaper clippings regarding the Hospital's Cup which was accessed in the uncatalogued archives of St. Brendan's Hospital when they were housed in Grangegorman. These records have recently been rehoused in the NAI but remained uncatalogued.
59. *Irish Examiner*, 29 January 1916.
60. *Skibbereen Eagle*, 17 March 1917.
61. Anon., 'Immediate need of doctors for the army' in *British Medical Journal*, 3015, no. 2 (1918), p. 417.
62. Winter, *The Great War*, p. 49.
63. Anon., 'Volunteers for medical service with the army' in *British Medical Journal*, 2798, no. 2 (1914), p. 343.
64. Abraham, *Surgeon's journey*, p. 133.
65. Whitehead, *Doctors in the Great War*, p. 91.
66. See Stuart Halifax, '"Over by Christmas": British popular opinion and the short war in 1914' in *First World War Studies*, 1, no. 2 (2010), pp. 103–121.
67. Alfred Keogh to Donald MacAlister, cited in Whitehead, *Doctors in the Great War*, p. 91.
68. Letter from Charles Brennan to the editor, *Evening Mail*, 29 March 1915.
69. Anon., 'Medical students and the war' in *British Medical Journal*, 2861, no. 2 (1915), p. 648.
70. Anon., 'Trinity College, Dublin and the war' in *British Medical Journal*, 2814, no. 2 (1914), p. 996.
71. McSwiney served until 1916 when he was forced to return to Ireland suffering from pneumonia. He died as a consequence of the disease. See Eugene McSwiney (RCPI, Kirkpatrick Index, TPCK/5/3).
72. Anon., 'Recruiting' in *British Medical Journal*, 2877, no. 1 (1916), p. 287.
73. Anon., 'Recruiting' in *British Medical Journal*, 2877, no. 1 (1916), p. 287.
74. *Irish Independent*, 22 September 1915.
75. Database of Irish medical officers in the British forces who served in the First World War.

76. Database of Irish medical officers in the British forces who served in the First World War.
77. Database of Irish medical officers in the British forces who served in the First World War.
78. Harrison, *The medical war*, p. 62.
79. Anon., 'Sir William Donovan' in *British Medical Journal*, 3841, no. 2 (1934), p. 335.
80. Papers of Colonel Sir William Donovan (WL, RAMC 523/4).
81. Whitehead, *Doctors in the Great War*, p. 83.
82. Vaughan and Fitzpatrick, *Irish historical statistics*, p. 246; Mary E. Daly, *The slow failure: Population decline and independent Ireland, 1920–73* (Madison, WI: University of Wisconsin Press, 2006), pp. 75–137.
83. Vaughan and Fitzpatrick, *Irish historical statistics*, p. 90.
84. Anon., 'Recruiting for the Naval and Military Medical Services' in *British Medical Journal*, 2877, no. 1 (1916), p. 617.
85. Diaries of J. P. Lynch, 5 August 1914 (WL, RAMC 453).
86. Diaries of Stafford Adye-Curran, 6 April 1915 (NLI, MS 34,393).
87. *Irish Times*, 28 April 1917.
88. Denis O'Donoghue (RCPI, Kirkpatrick Index, TPCK/5/3).
89. Jeffery, *Ireland and the Great War*, p. 12.
90. Jeffery, *Ireland and the Great War*, p. 12.
91. Ackroyd et al., *Advancing with the army*, p. 90.
92. Ackroyd et al., *Advancing with the army*, p. 91.
93. Susan M. Parkes, 'Higher education, 1793–1908' in W. E. Vaughan (ed.), *New history of Ireland VI: Ireland under the union 1: 1870–1921* (Oxford: Oxford University Press), p. 539.
94. Laura Kelly, *Irish medical education and student culture, c.1850–1950* (Liverpool: Liverpool University Press, 2017), pp. 9–27.
95. Kelly, *Irish medical education*, p. 10.
96. Parkes, 'Higher education', p. 567.
97. Greta Jones, *'Captain of these men of death': The history of tuberculosis in nineteenth and twentieth century Ireland* (New York: Rodopi, 2001), p. 13. In 1908, the Catholic University of Ireland's Medical School, established in 1855, was incorporated into UCD as its faculty of medicine.
98. Tomás Irish, *Trinity in war and revolution, 1912–1923* (Dublin: Royal Irish Academy, 2015), p. 100.
99. Crowther and Dupree, *Medical lives*, p. 23.
100. For instance, the Kirkpatrick Index, held in the RCPI, is chiefly concerned with Irish medical personnel who had careers in Ireland.
101. Laura Kelly, 'Migration and medical education: Irish medical students at the University of Glasgow, 1859–1900' in *Irish Economic and Social History*, 31, no. 1 (2012), p. 52.

102. Jane Leonard, 'The Catholic Chaplaincy' in Fitzpatrick (ed.), *Ireland and the First World War*, pp. 1–16; John Martin Brennan, 'Irish Catholic Chaplains in the First World War' (MPhil thesis, University of Birmingham, 2012), p. 119.

103. Diaries of Stafford Adye-Curran, 6 April 1915 (NLI, MS 34,393).

104. Diaries of Stafford Adye-Curran, 25 April 1915 (NLI, MS 34,393).

105. Diaries of Stafford Adye-Curran, 6 April 1915 (NLI, MS 34,393).

106. Diaries of J. P. Lynch, 22 October 1914 (WL, RAMC 453).

107. For more on the establishment of the college, see Harrison, *The medical war*, p. 7.

108. Report of Deputy Director of Medical Services, Irish Command, 26 January 1920 (TNA, Irish situation, 1914–22 collection, WO 35 179).

109. *Irish Times*, 20 November 1915.

110. Laura Dooney, 'Trinity College and the war' in Fitzpatrick (ed.), *Ireland and the First World War*, p. 41.

111. Dooney, 'Trinity College and the war', p. 41.

112. *Irish Times*, 10 May 1910.

113. *Irish Times*, 10 May 1910.

114. Harrison, *The medical war*, p. 16.

115. For a full insight into the workings of the 'medical machine', see Harrison, *The medical war*, pp. 16–64.

116. Diaries of J. P. Lynch, 3 August 1914 (WL, RAMC 453).

117. MacPherson, *History of the Great War*, p. 145.

118. Diaries of Stafford Adye-Curran, 6 April 1915 (NLI, MS 34,393).

119. Whitehead, *Doctors in the Great War*, p. 184.

120. Whitehead, *Doctors in the Great War*, p. 183.

121. Diaries of Richard George Hingston, 10 November 1914 (Trinity Manuscripts Library [hereafter TML], 10514).

122. Diaries of Stafford Adye-Curran, 17 April 1915 (NLI, MS 34,393).

123. Diaries of Stafford Adye-Curran, 20 April 1915 (NLI, MS 34,393).

124. CMWC minute book, 9 August 1916 (TNA, MH 47/162).

125. Eugene Ryan to his wife, 16 August 1915 cited in Ryan (ed.), *Haig's medical officer*, p. 102.

126. Diaries of Stafford Adye-Curran, 5 April 1915 (NLI, MS 34,393).

127. Diaries of Stafford Adye-Curran, 12 April 1915 (NLI, MS 34,393).

128. For more on shell shock, see Bourke, 'Effeminacy, ethnicity and the end of trauma', pp. 57–69; Joanna Bourke, 'Shell-shock, psychiatry and the Irish soldier during the First World War' in Adrian Gregory and Senia Paseta (eds.), *Ireland and the Great War: A war to unite us all* (Manchester: Manchester University Press, 2002), pp. 155–171; Edgar Jones and Simon Wessely, *Shell shock to PTSD: Military psychiatry from 1900 to the Gulf War* (New York: Psychology Press, 2005); Peter Leese,

*Shell shock: Traumatic neurosis and the British soldiers of the First World War* (Basingstoke: Palgrave Macmillan, 2002); Ben Shephard, *A war of nerves: Soldiers and psychiatrists, 1914–44* (London: Pimlico, 2002).

129. Bourke, 'Effeminacy, ethnicity and the end of Trauma', p. 58.

130. Lieutenant-General Sir Charles Burtchaell, 'Disease as affecting success in the war' in *Transactions of the Royal Academy of Medicine in Ireland*, xxxvii (1920), p. 540.

131. Diaries of Richard George Hingston, 13 May 1918 (TML, 10514).

132. Gordon, 'The Great European War', p. 28.

133. Whitehead, *Doctors in the Great War*, p. 190.

134. Diaries of J. P. Lynch, 22 August 1914 (WL, RAMC 453).

135. Diaries of J. P. Lynch, 26 August 1914 (WL, RAMC 453).

136. Henry Moore (RCPI, Kirkpatrick Index, TPCK/5/3).

137. Diaries of Stafford Adye-Curran, 21 April 1915 (NLI, MS 34,393).

138. Diaries of Stafford Adye-Curran, 31 May 1915 (NLI, MS 34,393).

139. Diaries of Stafford Adye-Curran, 24 April 1915 (NLI, MS 34,393).

140. Diaries of Stafford Adye-Curran, 25 April 1915 (NLI, MS 34,393).

141. Diaries of Stafford Adye-Curran, 30 May 1915 (NLI, MS 34,393).

142. Harrison, *The medical war*, p. 22.

143. Diaries of Stafford Adye-Curran, 7 June 1915 (NLI, MS 34,393).

144. Diaries of Stafford Adye-Curran, 2 June 1915 (NLI, MS 34,393).

145. Diaries of Richard George Hingston, 10 November 1914 (TML, 10514).

146. Clear, 'Fewer ladies, more women', p. 162.

147. *Irish Independent*, 19 August 1914.

148. For details on individual assignments, see Yvonne McEwen, *It's a long way to Tipperary: British and Irish nurses in the Great War* (Dunfermline: Cualann Press, 2006), pp. 61–83.

149. Janet Watson, 'A sister's war: The diaries of Alice Slythe' in Alison S. Fell and Christine E. Hallett (eds.), *First World War nursing: New perspectives* (London: Taylor & Francis, 2013), pp. 103–122.

150. Black, *King's nurse, beggar's nurse*, p. 84.

151. Black, *King's nurse, beggar's nurse*, p. 86.

152. Black, *King's nurse, beggar's nurse*, p. 86.

153. MMM, *A dream to follow*, p. 7.

154. Albert MacKinnon, *Malta: The nurse of the Mediterranean* (London: Hodder & Stoughton, 1916).

155. Clear, 'Fewer ladies, more women', p. 162.

156. Fell and Hallett, 'Introduction' in Fell and Hallett (eds.), *First World War nursing*, p. 7.

157. Black, *King's nurse, beggar's nurse*, p. 92.

158. Black, *King's nurse, beggar's nurse*, p. 92.

159. Black, *King's nurse, beggar's nurse*, p. 92.

160. MMM, *A dream to follow*, p. 10.
161. Marie Martin to her mother, 28 October 1915, cited in MMM, *A dream to follow*, p. 10.
162. Black, *King's nurse, beggar's nurse*, p. 93.
163. Black, *King's nurse, beggar's nurse*, p. 95.
164. For more on Anti-German sentiment in the First World War in Britain, see Panikos Panayi, 'Anti-German riots in London during the First World War' in *German History*, 7, no. 2 (1989), pp. 184–203. Other examples of Irish doctors displaying anti-German sentiment include Diaries of Stafford Adye-Curran, 25 June 1915 (NLI, MS 34,393); Postcards from Doran of Dublin to his family in Ireland while serving with the Royal Army Medical Corps (hereafter RAMC) in France (NLI, MS 24,581).
165. Diaries of Stafford Adye-Curran, 5 June 1915 (NLI, MS 34,393).
166. Diaries of J. P. Lynch, 29 August 1914 (WL, RAMC 453).
167. Diaries of J. P. Lynch, 27 November 1914 (WL, RAMC 453).
168. Diaries of J. P. Lynch, 27 November 1914 (WL, RAMC 453).
169. Draft letter by Sir Henry Rawlinson, 2 July 1916 (WL, RAMC 739/16).
170. Myles Dungan, *Distant drums: Irish soldiers in Foreign Armies* (Belfast: Appletree Press, 1993), p. 67.
171. Jane Leonard, 'The reaction of Irish Officers in the British Army to the Easter Rising of 1916' in Hugh Cecil and Peter Liddle (eds.), *Facing Armageddon: The First World War experienced* (Barnsley: Pen and Sword Military, 1996), p. 262.
172. Diaries of Richard George Hingston, 17 May 1916 (TML, 10514).
173. Tyquin, *Little by little*, p. 130.
174. Peter Rees, *The other Anzacs: nurses at war, 1914–1918* (Melbourne: Vision Australia Information Library Service, 2011), p. 211.
175. By 1929, 1484 Military Crosses in total had been awarded to members of the RAMC for their service in the conflict and Irish medical personnel featured heavily in honours lists. See J. S. G. Blair, *Centenary history of the medical corps, 1898–1998* (Edinburgh: Scottish Academic Press, 1998), p. 155.
176. Diaries of Richard George Hingston, 22 September 1916 (TML, 10514).
177. Diaries of J. P. Lynch, 1 August 1914 (WL, RAMC 453).
178. Diaries of Stafford Adye-Curran, 8 April 1915 (NLI, MS 34,393).
179. Diaries of Richard George Hingston, 26 July 1916 (TML, 10514).
180. Diaries of Stafford Adye-Curran, 5 June 1915 (NLI, MS 34,393).
181. Letter from Thomas Gibbon to his brother, 9 October 1914 (WL, RAMC/535).
182. Database of Irish medical officers in British forces who served in the First World War—based on a sample of 1000 doctors.

183. For more information on RAMC experiences in these areas, see Harrison, *The medical war*, pp. 16–64.
184. Harrison, *The medical war*, p. 7.
185. Charles Dalton (RCPI, Kirkpatrick Index, TPCK/5/3).
186. William Gordon Cummings (RCPI, Kirkpatrick Index, TPCK/5/3).
187. Harrison, *The medical war*, p. 195.
188. Bertram Letts (RCPI, Kirkpatrick Index, TPCK/5/3).
189. Harrison, *The medical war*, p. 234.
190. Reginald Holmes (RCPI, Kirkpatrick Index, TPCK/5/3).
191. Whitehead, *Doctors in the Great War*, p. 181.

# CHAPTER 4

# The First World War and Hospitals in Ireland, 1914–1918

'The necessity for additional hospital beds in Ireland was early recognised, and efforts were made to provide suitable accommodation. This was found to be a matter of great difficulty'.[1]

From 1914 to 1918, the RAMC's casualty evacuation system extended beyond the national borders that enclosed the battlefields of the Eastern and Western Fronts. Following extensive pre-war consultation between Sir Henry Wilson, Director of Military Operations and the Director General of the Army Medical Services, Launcellotte Gubbins, the RAMC decided that it would transport sick and wounded soldiers to Britain for treatment. Casualties were to be evacuated from ports near the front-lines to Britain by specially designed hospital ships and then distributed to military hospitals throughout the region. This was a significant movement away from the traditional method of wartime casualty treatment. In previous conflicts, the British Army medical services claimed that men transported home for treatment were unlikely to return to the battle-fields.[2] Nonetheless, the medical disasters of the Boer Wars encouraged the RAMC to consider a new approach to casualty dispersal.[3]

At the start of the First World War, the RAMC conceded that accommodation within Britain's military hospitals, similar to many other European regions, was inadequate for a large-scale conflict.[4] In August 1914, approximately 150 military hospitals were scattered throughout Britain. Most of these hospitals were small institutions that could cater

© The Author(s) 2019     93
D. Durnin, *The Irish Medical Profession and the First World War*,
Medicine and Biomedical Sciences in Modern History,
https://doi.org/10.1007/978-3-030-17959-5_4

to minimal numbers of soldiers—only ten of the 150 institutions had over 250 beds. In his official history of the British Army medical services of the First World War, William MacPherson estimated that military hospitals had provided about 7000 beds prior to August 1914.[5] It was therefore necessary for the RAMC to expand its hospital infrastructure to cope with the large number of soldiers that they expected to return to Britain for treatment. As part of a complex expansion programme, the RAMC authorised the extension of the number of existing military hospitals throughout the course of the war; twenty-three new territorial force general hospitals opened and new military hospitals were constructed or installed in existing buildings. The RAMC also decided to incorporate existing Irish military hospitals into the casualty evacuation system.[6]

By 1914, Ireland was home to several military hospitals situated in various cities, including Belfast, Cork and Dublin. These institutions became part of the RAMC's First World War casualty evacuation process. From 1914 to 1918, hospital ships transported approximately 20,000 soldiers—primarily those from Ireland—from the battlefields back to Ireland and the RAMC, Irish Command, distributed them among these hospitals.[7] Based on the findings of Surgeon General Louis Edward Anderson, Deputy Director of Medical Services (DDMS) of RAMC Irish Command, it was claimed in the DDMS' 1920 report that Ireland's military hospitals were inadequately prepared to cope with the demands of war. Richard Ford, Anderson's successor, noted that 'the necessity for additional hospital beds in Ireland, as elsewhere, was early recognised and efforts were made to provide suitable accommodation'.[8] Consequently, the RAMC authorised a complete overhaul of Ireland's military hospitals.

The RAMC also reached an agreement with more than forty civilian hospitals, located primarily in Belfast, Cork and Dublin, to provide accommodation and medical treatment for soldiers.[9] These hospitals were voluntary institutions, which relied on income garnered from public subscription schemes and donations.[10] One notable exception to the voluntary model was the state-funded Grangegorman asylum, which admitted soldiers from 1915 onwards. Existing studies of individual hospitals have detailed the wartime experience of Ireland's civilian hospitals and the treatment given to soldiers, which, while useful, tend to adopt an approach that is positivistic and descriptive rather than analytical.[11] Unlike those studies, this chapter is not concerned with the medical care soldiers received within hospitals and there is potential for future study here. Instead, it will examine the expansion of Ireland's military hospitals and assess the impact the conflict had on Ireland's civilian medical infrastructure, focusing on the civilian hospital system and specialist institutions. Moreover, this chapter will ask whether the involvement of civilian hospitals in the war affected hospital provision for civilians during the war years, thus adding to the debates raised by Winter on civilian healthcare and war.[12] As the RAMC altered its casualty dispersal system in 1916, when the corps decided to treat more soldiers near the front, this chapter is divided into two distinct periods—1914 to 1916 and 1917 to 1918—to explore whether the changes to the wider casualty dispersal process affected Irish hospitals.[13]

## CASUALTY EVACUATION SYSTEM, 1914–1916

Approximately three months after the declaration of war, wounded soldiers arrived on hospital ships in Ireland. On 26 October 1914, the *H.M.H.S. Oxfordshire*, built by Belfast-based Harland and Wolff, docked at Queenstown Harbour, County Cork. The luxury cruise liner, which military authorities had converted into a fully equipped hospital ship, was the first Great War vessel to arrive in Ireland. The *Oxfordshire* had travelled from the French port of Boulogne, the home of the RAMC's British Expeditionary Force Base Hospital, to Queenstown carrying 697 non-commissioned men and officers from several Irish and non-Irish regiments. This included the Connaught Rangers, Leinster Regiment and Royal Welsh Fusiliers. Following its arrival in Cork, a crowd of waiting local and national press boarded the ship.

Conditions on board the ships used to transport the wounded had come in for heavy criticism from doctors, military personnel and the press throughout the war. Following battles in several locations, most notably in Gallipoli, Basra and East Africa, the British Army medical services used regular transport vessels to evacuate soldiers requiring medical treatment and these ships were strongly condemned as overcrowded and unhygienic. Sir Victor Horsely, a surgeon in the RAMC, described the hospital ships used to transport the soldiers in Mesopotamia Campaign as 'foul store barges'.[14] The hospital ships that docked in Ireland between 1914 and 1916, however, were fully converted vessels designed solely for the transport of patients.[15] Newspaper reports and Pathé newsreel reveal that these ships were generally well equipped and the

*Oxfordshire* garnered universal praise from those who inspected the liner in Cork. The *Irish Times* reported:

> The Oxfordshire has long and spacious sick wards, where there were numbers of soldiers, most of whom were in bed whilst others were merely stretched on couches, carefully bandaged up, all of who were carefully attended to by a regiment of Red Cross nurses and fed with a first-rate menu of piping hot Irish stew, which they apparently relished. The sick soldiers' wards were of immense length and breadth, with plenty of ventilation and scrupulously clean. There were hundreds of small bedsteads within measurable distance of each other. Each one was occupied by a wounded soldier … it would be no exaggeration to say that there is not in Ireland a shore hospital equipped in a more admirable manner for wounded than the liner Oxfordshire.[16]

While this report may have overstated the quality of the conditions on the *Oxfordshire*, it provided some details on the structure and design of the hospital ship. Studies of the design of hospitals in the early twentieth century have found that architects, in association with hospital authorities, placed considerable importance on several design features, most notably ventilation and large wards.[17] The design of the *Oxfordshire* conversion—long accommodation areas, high ceilings and focus on ventilation—was clearly influenced by contemporary theories on the layout of hospitals during the late nineteenth and early twentieth centuries.

Once the *Oxfordshire* docked and members of the press had completed their tour, the RAMC offloaded patients onto two ambulance trains provided by the Great Southern and Western and Great Northern Railways. The railway companies converted these trains especially for the war, similar to the hospital ships, and paid particular attention to ventilation, lighting, and lavatory provision. Engineers lined the surgery car floor with zinc and deliberately rounded the corners in the carriages to assist with cleaning.[18] Each train accommodated approximately 130 soldiers. Britain's ambulance trains usually comprised of regular carriages in addition to those converted into pharmacies, kitchens and wards for injured soldiers confined to stretchers.[19] The Great Southern and Western Railway designed ambulance trains in a similar fashion. The first Irish ambulance train consisted of:

> five wards, each fitted with twenty cots in two tiers. These ward cars were converted from the company's standard 50 feet parcel vans, with the addition of end gangways, giving communication with a pharmacy car in

the centre. This latter car was also altered from a 50 feet van, and is sub-divided by means of suitable divisions into a surgery, pharmacy, linen stores, office for medical officers, etc., and provided with the necessary receptacles for drugs, bandages, and nursing utensils, and requirements … The various compartments are reached from a corridor, wide enough to accommodate a stretcher, a sliding door being provided in the partition to allow a patient to be carried into the treatment room sideways.[20]

There was also additional accommodation for medical personnel that catered for two doctors and two nurses. Nurses from the British Red Cross and St. John's Ambulance (SJA) initially staffed Irish hospital trains but this arrangement was discontinued during the war when military medical personnel took charge.[21]

In the early stages of the war, large crowds frequently assembled at railway stations to welcome the wounded, demonstrating support for the soldiers.[22] In October 1914, the *Irish Times* reported that large numbers had gathered at Cork City railway terminus. They included an official welcoming committee comprising medical men and prominent citizens. Local women presented the soldiers with newspapers, refreshments and cigarettes as they arrived on the platform.[23] Others provided assistance by gathering a convoy of motorcars to assist the RAMC with the transportation of soldiers from the station to nearby hospitals. The 697 soldiers that arrived in Cork were then sent to military and civilian hospitals in Dublin (326); Cork (250); Limerick (50); Fermoy (25); Waterford (20); Youghal (16) and Buttevant (10).[24]

Less than two weeks after its arrival in Cork, the *Oxfordshire*, which had returned to Boulogne to collect another contingent of approximately 700 sick and wounded, travelled to Dublin. Most of the soldiers on board had been wounded in the Battle of Messines, Belgian West Flanders, which took place in October 1914. Members of the Connaught Rangers, who had been in India for seven years prior to their involvement in the battles in France, were among the arrivals. This was their first visit to their native land in almost a decade.[25] At the Dublin docks to oversee the arrival of the wounded were some of the country's most eminent medical personnel including Dr. John Lumsden, Deputy Commissioner SJA. Lumsden had extensive medical and administrative experience and played a key role in the RAMC's casualty dispersal process in Ireland for the duration of the war. Lumsden was an MO at the Guinness Brewery from 1894 to 1940, as well as visiting physician to Mercer's Hospital from 1897 to 1939. In 1903, he founded the St. James's Gate Division of the SJA and using his influence at Guinness', he encouraged a significant number of the brewery's employees to enlist. When war broke out, military authorities accepted Lumsden's offer that his SJA brigade would manage the transport of the wounded in Ireland.[26]

Lumsden's SJA brigade was part of a network of military and voluntary organisations, established especially for the duration of the war, which controlled the First World War casualty dispersal process in Ireland. On the outbreak of conflict, organisations such as the British Red Cross Society in Ireland immediately pledged to assist the RAMC in their work. In September 1914, the Dublin Branch of the British Red Cross entered into an agreement with Lumsden's SJA Brigade to work together for the duration of the war. This agreement was made a month before a similar one was reached between the Red Cross and SJA in London.[27] The speed with which the voluntary groups in Ireland cooperated and offered their assistance suggests that there was complete unity among them but this was not the case.

Political division caused a split among the Irish Red Cross detachments and had considerable bearing on the First World War casualty dispersal process in Ireland. Lady Aberdeen, patron of the Red Cross in Dublin, had a fractious relationship with unionists who disapproved of her husband's—Lord Aberdeen, Lord Lieutenant of Ireland—support for Irish home rule.[28] In October 1914, a private letter written by Lady Aberdeen and sent to the editor of the *Freeman's Journal*, was leaked to two weekly papers—the nationalist *Sinn Féin* and the socialist *Irish Worker*.[29] In the letter, Aberdeen complained about unionist involvement in the Red Cross: 'I am afraid there is a bit of a plot amongst Unionists to capture the Red Cross Society in Ireland, and to run it in such a way from London, and through County Lieutenants and Deputy Lieutenants that it will be unacceptable to the Irish volunteer people'.[30] In response to the publication of the letter, Denis Pack-Beresford, Honorary Secretary of the British Red Cross Society in Dublin, requested that Aberdeen publicly disavow the authenticity of the letter due to 'the serious effect likely to be produced by this letter upon the work of our branch and upon that of the other branches throughout Ireland'.[31] Aberdeen replied that it was 'entirely unsuitable' for her to discuss the matter and she refused to renounce the letter.[32] Consequently, the Red Cross Branch in Ulster decided to act independently of the branches outside of the province resulting in a fractured casualty clearing system that operated independently north and south;

detachments of the British Red Cross in the north had little contact with those in the south.

This created a problem because the Red Cross had a significant role in casualty dispersal in Ireland. While the RAMC maintained control over the distribution of casualties, it was the voluntary groups that undertook the practical work of dispersal. Representatives of the British Red Cross Society noted that in Ireland, unlike Great Britain, voluntary organisations were entirely responsible for carrying out the casualty dispersal process.[33] Lumsden was a pivotal figure and guided the Red Cross and SJA in their duties. Additional assistance was received from the Royal Irish Automobile Club, an association formed in 1901 to further and promote interest in automobiles in Ireland.[34] Members of the automobile club provided vehicles to the SJA and the Red Cross to transport patients from the docks to the local hospitals. In addition, with financial support from the Red Cross, the automobile club constructed eighteen ambulances to assist in the process.[35] The two ambulance trains that were converted by the railway companies transported soldiers destined for institutions outside of Dublin—one train conveyed the wounded to Belfast station while the other was used to transfer men to Cork City, the Curragh Military Camp in County Kildare and the other military hospitals situated in the south of Ireland.[36]

An intricate network of voluntary organisations thus emerged in Ireland as a result of the First World War. For the remainder of the conflict, the majority of hospital ships arriving in Ireland docked in Dublin and the voluntary groups repeated the casualty dispersal process on each occasion. It is unsurprising that the RAMC transported the sick and wounded soldiers primarily to Dublin. Aside from its location, the city had a well-developed network of hospitals that was further strengthened by the opening of the King George V Military Hospital at Arbour Hill in 1914.[37]

## Irish Military Hospitals

As part of their wartime strategy, the RAMC expanded Irish military hospitals and this was fundamental to the treatment of returning soldiers to Ireland. Abel-Smith has established that in Britain, the RAMC expanded and improved hospital facilities for military patients by taking control of various workhouses, schools and lunatic asylums and converting them into centres for the treatment of sick and wounded soldiers.[38] Benefactors and philanthropic movements throughout Britain assisted the RAMC by providing approximately 5000 buildings, including stately homes, for use as hospitals.[39] Consequently, in Britain, permanent military hospitals accounted for only eight per cent of the total accommodation for these soldiers requiring medical treatment.[40] In contrast, while the RAMC hoped to follow a similar programme of development in Ireland, it ultimately proved too difficult. Many of the buildings that the Irish division of the RAMC had originally identified as appropriate sites for military hospitals or wards, including many workhouses and country houses, were 'either difficult to access or not provided with a water supply or satisfactory sewage system'.[41] As a result, military hospitals in Ireland accounted for forty-five per cent of total accommodation for soldiers returned for treatment; a much larger proportion than in Britain.[42] In total, the number of beds in Irish military hospitals grew from approximately 750 in 1914 to a peak of 4800 by the midpoint of the war.[43] Thus, the RAMC's military hospital expansion programme in Ireland was of the utmost importance to the domestic component of the wider casualty clearing process.

To assist in the dispersal of soldiers, the RAMC, Irish Command, effectively created and expanded three administrative districts based on brigades, divisions and Ireland's three main military hospitals—the Ulster Brigade in the north (Belfast), the Curragh and Dublin Brigade in the east (Dublin) and the 6th Division in the south (Cork). In the Eastern District, the King George V Hospital in Dublin was the RAMC's primary military hospital. The RAMC controlled the facility alongside the Royal Military Infirmary, which was located at nearby Montpelier Hill. The construction of the King George V hospital began in early 1914 and only one completed wing, with 102 beds, was finished in August. By December 1914, however, the main hospital building, which housed an operating theatre, laboratory, outbuildings, stores and an x-ray department had opened and was fully equipped.[44]

Prominent local medical personnel, who were experts in various specialist fields with positions in Dublin institutions, staffed the hospital alongside several RAMC men. RAMC, Irish Command, appointed Drs. Mathew Thompson and George Peacocks, Executive Officers for Clinical Medicine at the RCPI, as physicians. Dr. Henry Mason, a radiologist and skin specialist at Jervis Street Hospital, was employed as an x-ray specialist.[45] VAD nurses and members of QAIMNSR provided essential support in the nursing roles. The hospital was thus staffed for the reception of soldiers who arrived in Dublin Port.

There were approximately 30,000 admissions to the King George V Hospital during the war and there were notable surges in admissions following major battles.[46] Forty per cent (4941) of cases admitted in 1915 entered the hospital between January and April following the key battles at Neuve-Chapelle in March 1915 and Ypres in April 1915. In 1916, total admissions peaked at 6540 following the battles of Gallipoli in January 1916 and Verdun in February 1916. The nature of the wounds and illnesses varied among those admitted. The significant number of ophthalmic experts employed at the King George V ensured that the RAMC sent soldiers, including non-Irish men, suffering from injuries or diseases of the eye to the hospital for treatment.[47] In an article printed in the *British Medical Journal* in 1917, James Barrett argued that the RAMC prioritised the treatment of military ophthalmic cases in several hospitals as failure to do so would render the sufferer incapable of returning to the battlefields.[48] Patients who required ophthalmic surgery not only benefited from the King George V staff's medical expertise but also from the newly constructed surgical facilities available at the hospital.

From 1914 to 1918, approximately 4000 operations, ranging from small procedures for superficial injuries to full amputations, took place in the hospital.[49] The trio of surgeons—Frederick Conway-Dwyer, Henry Stokes and Colonel W. Taylor   performed surgeries and divided responsibilities between them. Each had significant surgical experience. From 1907 to 1922, Conway-Dwyer was surgeon to the Richmond hospitals. Following his enlistment into the RAMC, the War Office granted him the rank of lieutenant colonel and he subsequently received a knighthood in 1921 in recognition of his wartime role.[50] Taylor was an experienced member of the RAMC[51] while Stokes, who had graduated with an MD from TCD in 1905, had undertaken surgical duties in several Dublin hospitals prior to the outbreak of war.[52]

Figure 4.1 shows the increase in the number of operations carried out in the hospital from 1914 to 1918. There was a significant rise in surgical procedures carried out at the hospital from 1916 onwards that was partly due to the increase in the number of soldiers the RAMC returned to Ireland for treatment. Approximately six hospital ships arrived in 1915, ten in 1916 and twenty-one in 1917.[53] However, this does not fully explain the increase, as the number of operations carried out at the hospital remained relatively high in 1918 despite the fall in the number of hospital ships docking in Ireland that year—only four arrived in 1918.[54]

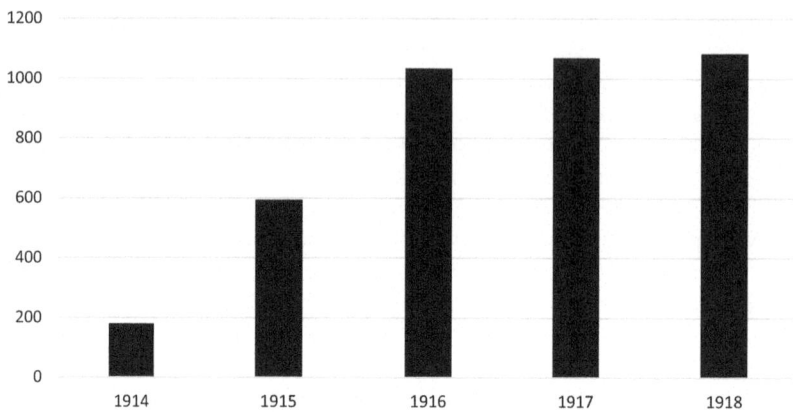

**Fig. 4.1** Number of operations carried out at King George V Hospital, 1914–1918 (*Source* Report of Deputy Director of Medical Services, Irish Command, 26 January 1920 [TNA, Irish situation, 1914–1922 collection, WO 35 179])

Rather, this surge in procedures is attributable to several other factors. Firstly, as Harrison has shown the RAMC altered the larger casualty clearing process from mid-1916. The majority of casualties in France and Belgium did not require transfer to domestic hospitals. Instead it was cheaper and more effective to treat them near the front.[55] It was only those who required prolonged treatment or more complex surgical procedures that were returned to domestic hospitals including those in Ireland. Therefore, while the number of hospital ships returning to Ireland declined in 1918, a larger percentage of soldiers admitted to the King George V Hospital required surgery.

Secondly, the RAMC appended an additional 300 beds to the hospital in 1915 and 1916 that increased the number of surgical cases that could be accommodated (Fig. 4.2). The expansion included the construction of thirty-eight hutments in the hospital grounds, which provided a further 300 beds in 1915. Lord Iveagh Edward Guinness, a prominent Irish businessman and philanthropist, funded the expansion.[56] Following the outbreak of brutal battles on the Western Front, including the Battle of the Somme in July 1916, and the subsequent increase in the number of hospital ships returning to Ireland, the RAMC further expanded accommodation at the hospital. By 1917, as wards were rearranged and hutments added, the number of beds available in the hospital had reached a peak of 921.

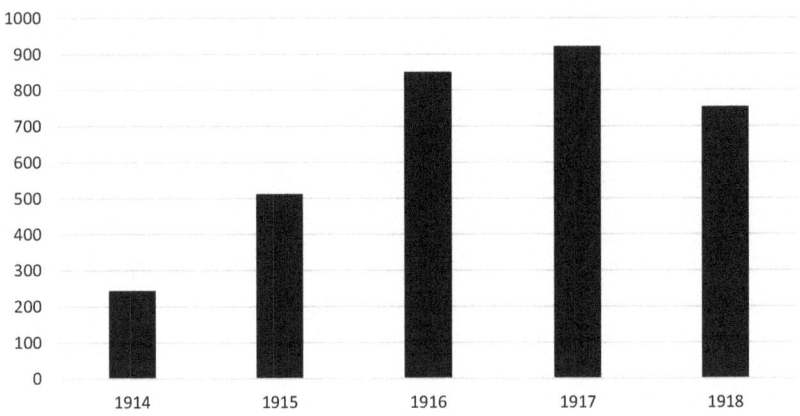

**Fig. 4.2**  King George V Hospital beds, 1914–1919 (*Source* Report of Deputy Director of Medical Services, Irish Command, 26 January 1920 [TNA, Irish situation, 1914–1922 collection, WO 35 179])

In the northern administrative district, approximately 150 soldiers who arrived on the first hospital ships in Cork and Dublin were immediately accommodated in the Military Hospital at Victoria Barracks, Belfast, and the Royal Victoria Hospital, Belfast, with less serious cases travelling to Downpatrick and Omagh.[57] Following the arrival of wounded soldiers into the region, the Ulster Volunteer Force (UVF), a military organisation founded in 1912 to oppose Home Rule in Ireland, offered to establish a hospital for the War Office in Belfast.[58] The War Office accepted the proposal. In November 1914, Lieutenant General Sir George Richardson, General Officer Commanding the UVF, launched a public appeal for funds to equip the hospital for approximately 100 soldiers in Belfast.[59] Sir Edward Carson, unionist and key figure in the founding of the UVF, supported the appeal and in a public letter, published in several newspapers, stated:

> this [establishing a hospital] will necessarily involve a great deal of outlay, and we must appeal to all friends of the Volunteers to help us in this most urgent duty … how can we better show our admiration and our gratitude than by making provision for the care of those who are daily adding lustre to our great traditions, and preserving for us the rights and liberties we so highly value?[60]

Having raised sufficient funds, the UVF established the hospital in Belfast's Exhibition Hall in the centre of the city. On 8 January 1915, the group officially presented the hospital to the War Office with Lady Carson performing the ceremonial opening of the institution. The UVF Hospital, a name retained by the hospital despite being under War Office control, became one of the primary hospitals in Ulster for the treatment of soldiers.[61]

Soldiers sent to the UVF hospital by the RAMC first arrived at the Belfast Railway Station. There, RAMC officers assessed the sick and injured and organised transport to the UVF hospital, an auxiliary hospital or one of the ten smaller military hospitals in the district. Some cases would be sent to an auxiliary hospital first, before being later transferred to the UVF Hospital.[62] As Fig. 4.3 demonstrates, between 1915 and 1917, the number of sick and wounded sent to Belfast increased and this forced the RAMC to expand the hospitals in the northern district. Within several months of its opening, the number of beds in the UVF Hospital had increased from 50 to 336.

The new wards were named in honour of notable politicians and committees including the Union Jack Committee and James Craig, a leader of the Ulster Unionist Party.[63] The corps also increased staff levels;

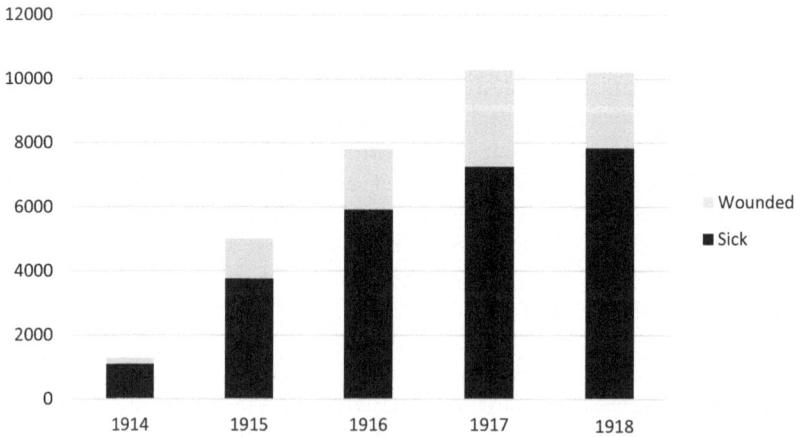

**Fig. 4.3** Sick and wounded soldiers transferred to RAMC northern district (*Source* Report of Deputy Director of Medical Services, Irish Command, 26 January 1920 [TNA, Irish situation, 1914–1922 collection, WO 35 179])

Captain I. A. Davidson, RAMC, a specialist in ophthalmology and diseases of the ear, nose and throat, joined the hospital in 1915, while Dr. Henry Lawrence McKisack, President of the Ulster Branch of the BMA, and temporary Lieutenant Colonel Thomas Myles, Surgeon to the King in Ireland, acted as consultant physician and consultant surgeon, respectively.[64]

As well as enhancing hospital facilities in the North, the RAMC also expanded military hospitals in their southern administrative district.[65] The successful distribution of the first group of casualties that arrived in Cork in October 1914 on the *Oxfordshire* demonstrated the effectiveness of military medical infrastructure in the region. Cork Military Hospital (CMH) was the primary military hospital in the southern administrative district. It was part of the Victoria Barracks, a long-standing military garrison, established by the British Army on the Old Youghal Road on the north side of Cork City in 1801. On the outbreak of war, the RAMC acquired three blocks of barrack rooms within the compound. This allowed the corps to extend the hospital and increase the number of beds from seventy-eight to 218 and to establish departments for the treatment of ophthalmic, muscle and dental complaints. In September 1917, the RAMC took over another block near the hospital and this provided a further fifty beds for less serious cases.[66]

Despite the increased number of beds, the CMH could not accommodate all the soldiers that arrived in Cork because of the number of sick and wounded sent to the city. Between 1914 and 1918, fourteen convoys of sick and wounded soldiers arrived in Cork from Dublin.[67] Like the dispersal programme established in Dublin and Belfast, the officer in charge of patient distribution in Cork relied on the smaller military hospitals located in the district to cater for the overflow.[68] These hospitals were situated in British military garrisons in the towns and cities of Buttevant, Fermoy, Limerick, Queenstown and Tipperary. Richard Ford, RAMC, Irish Command, subsequently stated in his post-war report that 'it soon became evident that this accommodation was insufficient for war conditions' and therefore certain improvements and expansions were carried out at the smaller hospitals as part of the nationwide hospital expansion programme.[69] The RAMC increased the number of beds in Buttevant Hospital in County Cork from sixteen to 137—converting two dining halls and using the 'J' Block in the barracks to house the new beds. Fermoy Military Hospital, also in County Cork, underwent a complete overhaul of its facilities—a new wing was added that consisted of three general wards, one officer's ward and an operating theatre. New accommodation huts were added and the number of beds increased from sixty-five to 210.[70] At Limerick Military Hospital, Limerick City, the RAMC converted a barrack room and a nurse's duty room into accommodation for wounded soldiers, increasing the number of hospital beds in the institution from twenty-six to seventy-two. In total, hospital accommodation for soldiers in the Southern Administrative District military hospitals increased by approximately 370 per cent from 1914 to 1918.[71] The significant increase in bed capacity for military cases, evident throughout the three Irish districts, indicates the extent to which the First World War prompted a major expansion of military medical infrastructure in Ireland.

The British Red Cross and several Irish civilian hospitals largely provided the remainder of the accommodation to treat soldiers. On 1 December 1914 delegates of the British Red Cross, Dublin Branch, met in the Mansion House, Dublin, to discuss a scheme to convert part of Dublin Castle, the seat of British rule in Ireland, into a hospital for the accommodation of 450 wounded soldiers.[72] According to Sir Thomas Myles, a key supporter of the plan, the scheme had several strengths: firstly, Dublin Castle was situated in the middle of Dublin, close to the administrative centre of the RAMC and a convenient location for the medical personnel attached to it; secondly, none of the money raised through public subscriptions for the hospital would be spent on construction works, as the Board of Public Works would carry out the necessary structural changes; finally, the Red Cross believed that the castle would be fully operational within a short timeframe.[73]

Following the December meeting in the Mansion House, the Red Cross Society established a committee of management for the hospital and its membership reveals that several prominent members of Irish society were instrumental in organising healthcare for soldiers. The committee included the Marchioness of Aberdeen (Chair); Sir John Lynch (vice-chairman), a solicitor for the Women's National Health Association; William M. Murphy (Chairman of the Finance Committee), who was notorious for his role in the 1913 Lockout,[74] and the presidents of the RCSI and RCPI. The Red Cross donated a significant financial endowment to the Board of Public Works to enable them to carry out the necessary alterations to Dublin Castle.

A number of problems threatened to derail the Dublin Castle conversion. Firstly, supporters of the scheme were concerned that Lady

Aberdeen's involvement in the project would discourage donations from unionists. In a letter to the *Irish Times* encouraging support for the scheme, Thomas Myles noted that 'the class of people in Dublin and throughout Ireland which in the past has subscribed most generously to charitable objects is completely out of sympathy with the principal promoters of the scheme under discussion'.[75] He proposed that the public ignore these concerns and argued that everyone involved with the scheme should:

> practise a little self-sacrifice and self-effacement. Let us no longer be Montagues or Capulets, but let us think only, on these cold, wet, and stormy nights, of our brave soldiers, heroes, nameless too often, lying in the frozen sludge of the trenches, giving their lives for us without a murmur, enduring with stoical fortitude atrocious suffering; and let us all pledge ourselves that, with God's help, we shall each and every one do his share.[76]

Secondly, a disagreement between the Red Cross and the War Office over the suitability of the castle's rooms delayed the hospital's opening. The War Office were concerned about the sanitary arrangements within the castle and the suitability of the rooms chosen by the Red Cross to convert into wards.[77] The War Office refused to send soldiers to the castle until additional alterations were carried out and, as a result, the Red Cross spent twice the amount of money than was originally envisioned on the hospital's establishment.[78]

The development of a positive public image for the hospital was crucial to its fundraising efforts. The hospital's committee was concerned that the War Office's apprehension about the hospital had dented public enthusiasm for the project and thus had damaged subscription rates.[79] In an attempt to curb negative reactions, the committee published a pamphlet which emphasised that 'there was no ground at any time for such apprehension, and that the Castle Hospital is now a hospital in being – only waiting patients to embark on its beneficent career'.[80] In a further offensive, the presidents of the RCPI and RCSI co-authored a letter, published as another pamphlet and exclusively concerned with the Dublin Castle Hospital, in which they reassured the public that

> before signing the letter asking the public to subscribe funds for converting Dublin Castle into a temporary hospital, we carefully inspected the building first as to accommodation, and second, as to sanitary conditions.

> In this inspection we had the assistance of Sir Charles Cameron, several
> medical members of the Committee of the City of Dublin branch of the
> British Red Cross Society, and a representative of the Board of Works. We
> were satisfied that the castle was suitable for the suggested purpose and
> that the sanitation was perfect.[81]

Sir Charles Cameron, Dublin's Chief MO, was the city's leading authority on sanitation.[82] In mentioning his inspectoral role, the presidents
provided extra assurance to potential subscribers that the Dublin Castle
Red Cross Hospital was suitable for patients.

Having addressed these public concerns and attempting to assure
them that the hospital was fit for use, the hospital committee focused on
fundraising and equipping and staffing the institution. In doing so, the
committee demonstrated the highly collaborative nature of the work that
was necessary to ensure the establishment and continued running of a
temporary hospital for military patients. Any concerns that the involvement of Lady Aberdeen would negatively affect subscriptions were soon
put to rest as the committee quickly established a subscription list worth
£4800.[83] The Red Cross Society, Dublin Branch, also collected funds
from several private philanthropists.[84] At a meeting of the Women's
National Health Association of Ireland, Lady Aberdeen, in her capacity as president of the group, asked its members to help provide further
equipment and beds for the hospital and several of those at the meeting
made 'definite offers of help'.[85] Ultimately, the institution was equipped
with donated beds and medical equipment. Medical personnel from
local civilian hospitals staffed the institution. On 7 December 1914, the
Dublin Castle Red Cross Hospital Committee requested that the medical
boards of each clinical hospital in the Dublin area nominate a surgeon
and physician to undertake work in the hospital and this arrangement
continued for the duration of the war.[86]

The establishment of the hospital in Dublin Castle increased the number
of medical institutions in Ireland that admitted soldiers and this was important for the British Military medical services, given the increasing number
of men that were returning for treatment. According to MacPherson, the
number of sick and wounded soldiers transported to Britain and Ireland
for treatment increased from approximately 73,000 in 1914 to a peak of
700,000 in 1917 (Fig. 4.4).[87] This increase was the result of the growing
number of casualties evacuated by army medical services from other theatres of war, including Gallipoli, Salonika and East Africa.[88]

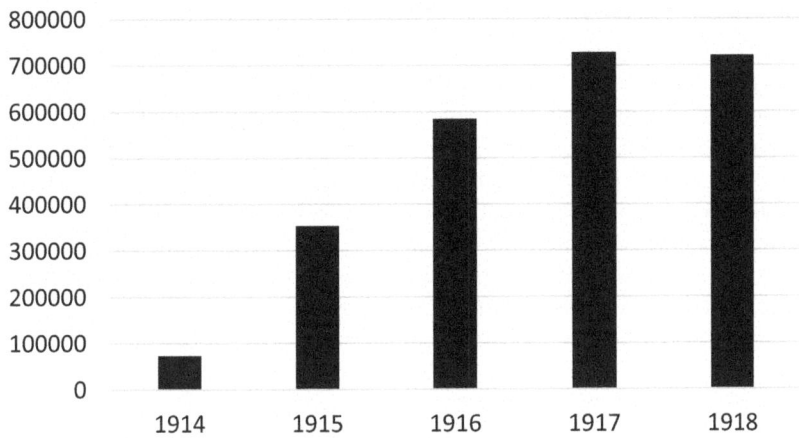

**Fig. 4.4** Number of wounded soldiers arriving in Britain from the battlefields, 1914–1918 (*Source* MacPherson, *History of the Great War*, vol. I, p. 372)

To cope with the numbers returning, RAMC, Irish Command, also requested civilian hospitals in their three administrative districts to help.[89] This had a significant impact on the Irish civilian hospital system.

## CIVILIAN HOSPITALS, 1914–1916

At the start of the war, Dublin was home to thirty-two hospitals that provided 3200 beds.[90] Eleven of the hospitals received small amounts of government funding while the remainder were wholly voluntary institutions established during the eighteenth and nineteenth centuries to cater to various religious and charitable groups.[91] Most of these hospitals treated patients free of charge and relied on state and philanthropic support to remain open.[92] By the end of August 1914, Surgeon General Anderson, RAMC, Irish Command, had contacted every hospital in Dublin requesting them to inform him whether their hospital could accommodate sick and wounded soldiers and, if so, the number of beds which would be available and their terms and conditions.[93]

Most hospital governors responded positively. The Meath Hospital governors agreed to set apart thirty beds for soldiers. In addition, the governors announced that they would place land at the disposal of the military authorities to establish a temporary building in case of emergency.[94] In total, twenty of Dublin's civilian hospitals, including the Adelaide, Jervis Street and Mater hospitals, provided accommodation for soldiers during the First World War. Another sixteen smaller institutions within the RAMC's eastern district provided convalescent facilities and the corps secured approximately 1200 additional civilian hospital beds in the northern and southern districts.[95] There was a clear classification between officers and men when it came to treatment.[96] The RAMC preferred to treat military officers in hospitals and wards that did not treat regular soldiers and thus acquired additional hospital facilities in Ireland for the officer class, including the ten-bed Fitzwilliam Street hospital in Dublin.[97]

The treatment of wounded soldiers in domestic civilian hospitals was a natural extension of the Irish medical professions' support for the British Army medical services during conflict. In addition, the War Office offered to pay a maintenance grant to hospitals for each soldier and this had the potential to alleviate the financial crisis that plagued many of the hospitals.[98] When offering beds for soldiers, the Meath Hospital governors informed the War Office that they would charge £1. 1s. per week for each occupied bed.[99] The governors also agreed to reserve unoccupied beds but did not agree on any form of remuneration with the War Office for this concession.

By the early twentieth century, Ireland's civilian hospitals were in a precarious financial position. Their overreliance on charitable donations made them susceptible to downturns in public financial support. In the years prior to the outbreak of the First World War, several of Dublin's civilian hospitals suffered financial hardship due to a significant fall in public donations and bequests.[100] According to William Martin Murphy, who was interviewed in 1913 by a Committee inquiring into the extension of medical benefit under the National Insurance Act to Ireland, 'only for people dying occasionally and leaving legacies the hospitals could not be kept up at all'.[101] The War Office's offer of payment for each soldier under treatment therefore appealed to hospital governors.

More importantly for the finances, the hospitals' acceptance of returning soldiers prompted an immediate rise in income from donations from philanthropic groups. On 11 December 1914, the British Red Cross Society, Dublin Branch, circulated a letter to every civilian hospital in Dublin announcing that they were considering giving a grant to the Dublin hospitals which treated wounded soldiers and enclosed a list of questions which they required the hospital governors to answer, including a query as to the number of beds available for wounded.[102] This was part of the society's wartime strategy in both Ireland and Britain—providing financial support to civilian hospitals for the purposes of establishing wards for soldiers within existing institutions rather than purchasing and equipping new buildings. The society argued that this was a better use of the money raised due to the considerable expense involved in building or establishing numerous new hospitals.[103]

From 1914 to 1918, Red Cross contributions were among the largest donations received by Ireland's hospitals. In most cases, the society covered the cost of furnishing whole wards with new beds and provided regular financial support towards the upkeep of these wards at later intervals. On 13 January 1915, for example, Sir Patrick Dun's Hospital accepted £75 from the Joint Committee of the British Red Cross Society and SJA Brigade as a contribution to the hospital's funds.[104] The society also covered the cost of equipment for the wards. In December 1915, the governors of the House of Industry Hospitals in Dublin requested that Thomas Myles, in his capacity as Lieutenant Colonel, encourage the War Office to cover the cost of a new x-ray machine needed for work on the wounded. Myles responded that the government only provided apparatus to military hospitals.[105] A week after this refusal, the governors received a letter from the Red Cross offering to cover the cost of the machine.[106]

Over the course of the war, hospital governors grew to rely on the society for financial support and it was not unusual for them to lodge direct requests with the organisation for financial aid. On 21 May 1915, for instance, the governors of the House of Industry Hospitals requested funds from the Red Cross to allow the institution to comply with an RAMC request to equip an extra thirty-six beds for wounded soldiers.[107] On 1 October 1915, the Red Cross sent £825 for seventy-five extra beds that had been installed. Similarly, on 8 October, the society sent £250 to the Royal City of Dublin Hospital to cover the maintenance cost of equipping the extra twenty-five beds provided by Lord Iveagh for the reception of soldiers.[108] In October 1915 alone, the Red Cross contributed approximately £2000 to Dublin's hospitals.[109]

Large donations not only came from philanthropic groups. A number of wealthy individuals also contributed to the hospitals' funds specifically to cover the cost of soldiers' care. Between 1914 and 1918, Lord Iveagh became one of the largest individual contributors to Dublin's civilian hospital network. Iveagh had a strong tradition of providing financial support to Irish medical services that assisted the British Army during conflicts. In 1900, he had funded the construction of a 100-bed hospital that Irish medical personnel established in South Africa to provide medical care to the soldiers participating in the Boer War.[110] He continued his philanthropic support during the First World War and contributed considerable financial assistance to domestic hospitals willing to admit soldiers. On 12 February 1915, the board of governors of the Royal City of Dublin Hospital informed the Red Cross, following a query from the society, that it would be able to provide an additional twenty-five new beds for soldiers. The governors estimated that the cost of the extra beds, fitted and ready for use, was approximately £10 each.[111] On 11 June 1915, the Red Cross replied that Iveagh had offered to cover the cost and the beds were delivered within two days.[112] Iveagh provided similar financial patronage to several other hospitals in the Dublin region throughout the war years.[113]

Over the course of the war, other high-profile contributors and members of the public donated to the hospitals through annual subscription schemes established by hospital governors. For example, Vicountess Powerscourt—Sybil Pleydell-Bouverie, wife of the Lord Lieutenant of Wicklow—donated one guinea per year to Sir Patrick Dun's Hospital for the purposes of maintaining a soldiers' ward.[114] Sir Patrick Duns' annual reports show that general members of the public also contributed to the war ward through the subscription scheme and 5s. was the most common subscription rate.[115]

Due to the increase in public donations and the considerable financial support from the British Red Cross and individual contributors, Dublin's civilian hospitals experienced a revival in income in comparison with the revenue received before the war. In December 1914, the Royal City of Dublin Hospital governors recorded an overall annual income of £2051 from subscriptions and donations compared to £1259 in the previous year. Income from paying patients also increased as the War Office contributed £1168 towards the cost of the soldiers' maintenance. Each civilian hospital in the Dublin district that received returning soldiers, and whose wartime financial records remain accessible, experienced a significant rise in income during the war years. Sir Patrick Dun's Hospital financial accounts provide a suitable example. As shown in Fig. 4.5, the hospital's income increased by approximately sixty per cent in 1915.

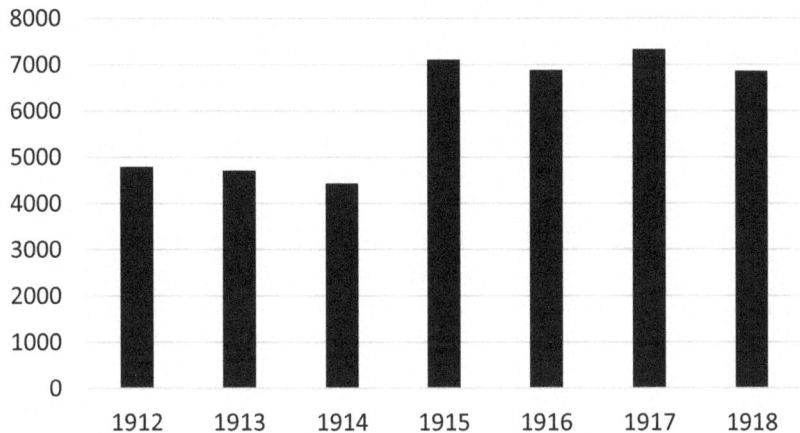

**Fig. 4.5**  Sir Patrick Dun's Hospital income, 1912–1918 (exclusive of bequests) (*Source* Sir Patrick Dun's Hospital Annual Reports, 1912–1918 [RCPI, PDH/1/1/6-7])

The hospital began admitting soldiers in the latter months of 1914 and it is understandable that the impact of the war on income levels in that year was minimal. As the conflict progressed, the hospital's financial position improved as donations, subscriptions and income from the War Office increased. The returns remained significantly high for the remainder of the war. Dun's hospital is an exemplar of broader trends and is largely representative of several other hospitals that admitted soldiers. Income at the Royal City of Dublin Hospital, for example, grew by forty per cent—from £6772 in 1913 to £9506 in 1915.[116]

While hospitals undoubtedly witnessed an improvement in their income levels during the war years, ultimately most suffered financially due to the rising costs associated with the conflict. As Stephen Broadberry has shown, the First World War encouraged the onset of inflation in Britain.[117] Martin Kitchen has unequivocally argued that while economic historians will continue to debate the long-term effects of war, there is no doubt that the conflict had a profound and shattering impact on economic life in the short term.[118] The financial effects of the war extended to Ireland as prices of daily goods, including fuel and food increased and this significantly raised the cost of hospital overheads.

Rising admission numbers, coupled with a significant increase in the price of daily supplies, multiplied hospital expenditure significantly. From 1914 to 1916, expenditure on medicines increased as supply slowed and the cost of drugs surged.[119] The RAMC established a depot of medical stores in Dublin in an attempt to counteract this problem. Hospitals obtained the drugs and dressings from local contractors, while staff at the depot organised the distribution of supplies to the various hospitals.[120] Traditionally, light and heat, and provisions for the maintenance of patients—food, surgical dressings and bandages—were a hospital's highest costs. Hospital governors usually entered into annual agreements with suppliers to provide items at a fixed price. Yet from 1915 onwards, hospital governors found themselves inundated with requests from suppliers to alter these agreements and increase the price due to the economic conditions. On 12 March 1915, for example, the Royal City of Dublin Hospital governors acceded to an appeal from Thomas Heiton and Company requesting an increase in the contract price of coal owing to 'the exceptional circumstances brought about by the war'.[121] At the Royal Victoria Hospital, Belfast, annual meeting, the treasurer reported an overall loss of more than £2000 for 1915 and noted that this was expected as 'it was known that prices of most supplies would be considerably increased owing to the war'.[122] In most cases, governors had little choice but to agree to suppliers' demands as other suppliers also increased prices. Table 4.1 and Fig. 4.6 charts the increasing expenditure at Sir Patrick Dun's Hospital between 1913 and 1918. Costs almost doubled during the war years, an inflationary trend that was replicated in other Irish hospitals.[123]

By early 1915, the governors of several Irish civilian hospitals had requested that the War Office increase their payment not only due to the rising costs but also because of the lack of soldiers in the wards. Hospital governors complained that they had reserved beds for military

**Table 4.1** Sir Patrick Dun's Hospital expenditure on provisions and light and heat, 1913–1918

|  | 1913 | 1914 | 1915 | 1916 | 1917 | 1918 |
|---|---|---|---|---|---|---|
| Provisions | £1035 | £1165 | £1489 | £1687 | £1907 | £2090 |
| Light and heat | £689 | £776 | £901 | £1001 | £1143 | £963 |

*Source* Sir Patrick Dun's Hospital Annual Reports, 1912–1918 (RCPI, PDH/1/1/6-7)

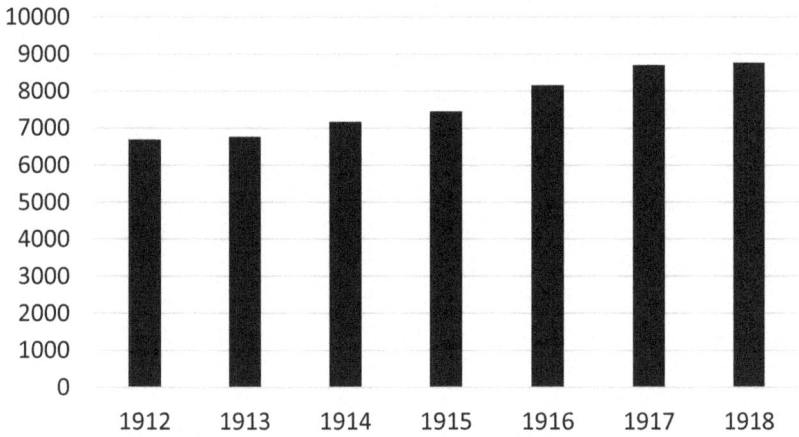

**Fig. 4.6** Sir Patrick Dun's Hospital expenditure, 1912–1918 (exclusive of building accounts) (*Source* Sir Patrick Dun's Hospital Annual Reports, 1912–1918 [RCPI, PDH/1/1/6-7])

patients but that more often than not, these beds remained empty. In these instances, the hospitals did not receive any payment. Dr. Steevens' Hospital in Dublin, for example, set aside sixty beds for wounded soldiers for 212 days. According to the hospital governors' method of calculations, this was a total offering of 12,720 available beds.[124] Of this number, only 3047 were occupied; 9673 remained unoccupied. Thus, as far as the governors were concerned, this was 'more than two-thirds, for which no payment was received'.[125] Hospital governors corresponded on the issue: the Meath hospital governors contacted both the British Hospitals' Association and the governors of several other hospitals, including the Royal City of Dublin Hospital to rally support.[126] Eventually, the hospital governors opted to enter into collective negotiations using the Hospital Board of Superintendence as an intermediary with the War Office. The Hospital Board of Superintendence, established in 1856, was a statutory body that inspected all Dublin hospitals in receipt of government funding.[127] On 4 January 1915, Dr. Richard Tobin, Secretary of the Hospital Board of Superintendence of Dublin Hospitals, informed the governors that he was endeavouring to secure the best possible financial terms for the hospitals.[128] Following negotiations, the War Office agreed to pay the governors an increased rate of 4*s.* per day, per occupied bed. The hospitals failed to reach an agreement with the War Office on payment for unoccupied beds, yet the governors agreed to continue to provide beds for soldiers.[129] In the RAMC's other districts, hospital rates largely varied from 2*s.* to 4*s.* per day. In September 1914, the Royal Victoria Hospital in Belfast decided to charge for soldiers what it cost to maintain them but by 1915, the hospital took direction from the British Hospitals' Association, who encouraged a uniform charge across all voluntary hospitals. By 1915, the hospitals' charges began to rise.[130]

While financial terms were a subject of continuous negotiation between Ireland's hospital governors and the War Office, both parties were seemingly content with the treatment of soldiers within the hospital wards. In the hospitals, governors ensured that the soldiers' beds were set apart from accommodation for civilians as per the agreement with the War Office. Several hospitals reorganised their institutions specifically to cater for the soldiers. For instance, the Meath Hospital dedicated one of the hospital's larger wards for the accommodation of soldiers thereby keeping the military patients together and separate from civilians.[131] Hospital governors took this agreement seriously. On 21 May 1915, for instance, the governors of the House of Industry Hospitals reprimanded medical staff for admitting civilians into the soldiers' ward.[132] On their admission to hospital, soldiers were also given a distinctive blue uniform to distinguish them from regular patients. As in Britain, soldiers were obliged to wear this uniform, even when they convalesced away from the hospital.[133]

While soldiers were distinct from civilians within the hospitals, the military and civilian patients' time in the wards appears to have been similar, albeit with some additional benefits for the soldier. Winter has argued that the conditions working-class soldiers witnessed in hospitals probably discouraged them to repeat the experience.[134] In contrast, according to Abel-Smith, soldiers admitted to civilian hospitals throughout Britain were usually well cared for—they were permitted to smoke in the wards, locals provided entertainment and supplies including car rides and newspapers.[135] There is little evidence to suggest that soldiers treated in Irish civilian hospitals were dissatisfied with the facilities. Staff treated soldiers well and provided them with several additional benefits compared to civilian patients because of the gifts donated by members of the public. On 11 December 1914, the Royal City of Dublin Hospital received several gifts from the public and various businesses for the soldiers. These included:

> two carcases of venison from the Phoenix Park herd of deer presented by the Office of Public Works; one copy of the Daily Express (Heroes Edition) [sic] presented daily to each soldier in the hospital by the proprietors of the Daily Express [sic]; special gifts of shirts and socks for each soldier, presented by the Ladies Field, London; the Irish Automobile Club offered to take the soldiers for motor drives as often as required; 60 Pheasants for the wounded, presented by Hon. Cosby G. Trench and Lord Inchiquin and large consignments of butter, presented by the Irish Creamery Manager's Association.[136]

Soldiers in hospitals across Ireland benefited from similar donations throughout the war. Hospital governors, aware of the public generosity towards those injured at war, often placed appeals in the newspapers for items required by the soldiers. On 11 June 1915, for instance, the Royal City of Dublin Hospital received six merlin chairs from the local Church of Ireland clergy following an appeal in the press for its wounded military patients.[137]

While hospital authorities were eager to ensure the comfort of a soldier's stay in hospital, ultimately, the RAMC wanted the wounded promptly returned to the battlefields. To achieve this, the War Office established an Irish branch of the Expeditionary Force Office (EFO) to manage soldiers in civilian hospitals. It dealt with issues related to pay and discipline among military patients and encouraged the swift return of soldiers' to active duty. Originally, the RAMC had planned to have the staff of the King George V Hospital undertake these duties but the EFO assumed the responsibilities due to the considerable workload of the hospital staff. A senior regular RAMC officer, assisted by a junior RAMC Officer and a Regimental Officer, staffed the medical wing of the Irish EFO.[138] An EFO officer visited several hospitals daily, examined patients, consulted with medical staff and compiled a list of patients who were to be discharged from each hospital to ensure that they were returned to duty as quickly as possible. Through consultations with the hospitals' medical staff, an EFO officer also determined the length of a soldier's stay in civilian hospitals; the shortest recorded stay in Sir Patrick Dun's Hospital, for example, was two days while the longest was 208 days.[139] In the Royal Victoria Hospital in Belfast, the shortest length of stay among the first contingent of wounded to arrive was seven days, while Private J. West of the Lincoln Regiment was in the hospital for 182 days.[140] It was almost impossible for the RAMC to overlook a soldier as EFO representatives visited each hospital approximately once a week.

Hospital medical staff did not always welcome the EFO officer's opinion on a soldiers' health and this was indicative of the doctors' wider resentment towards the extension of military supervision into their wards. As part of their wartime strategy, the War Office appointed two prominent Irish medical men—Sir Charles Ball and Thomas Myles—to serve as Ireland's consulting surgeons to the Army. Ball, similar to Myles, was an Honorary Surgeon to the King in Ireland and had acquired surgical experience in several Dublin hospitals throughout his career.[141] W. M. Russell, Deputy Director of Medical Services RAMC, Irish Command, outlined the duties of the two consulting surgeons in a circular sent to the auxiliary civilian hospitals in Ireland:

> They will be authorised to visit all official and voluntary institutions where there is wounded, to ensure that the best surgical assistance is being afforded. They will represent any shortcomings to you whether on the part of individuals or in the matter of stores or equipment, and in case of urgency will take such steps as the occasion demands. They will operate themselves in cases which they consider such a course desirable, and will advise others engaged in operation work. In general terms they will exercise supervision over the surgical work in connection with the military hospitals and other institutions in Ireland, in which wounded are treated, and will keep you informed of the results of their observations.[142]

Physicians and surgeons were angered by the War Office's insistence that Ball and Myles had, what the medical staff saw as, the right to criticise the work of members of the civilian medical profession and thus undermine the autonomy of hospitals and doctors. On 5 December 1914, the medical board of the Mater Misericordiae Hospital responded to the War Office insisting that they would not permit anyone other than a member of the hospital staff to supervise and criticise the treatment of, or to operate on, the patients under their care. The board emphasised that the staff of the Mater have given their 'service ungrudgingly to the wounded soldiers, officers and men, without thought of remuneration. Apparently, their action has not earned immunity from insult'.[143]

On the 11 December 1914, the Dublin Clinical Hospitals' Committee held a special meeting to discuss the Army's consulting surgeons. Charles Ball and Thomas Myles pre-empted this meeting and addressed the committee by letter to ease the concerns of their colleagues. In it, they explained that their duties included a general supervision of the arrangements made for the treatment of wounded soldiers in public and private institutions throughout Ireland. However, they stressed that they were well aware that the treatment received by wounded soldiers in the clinical hospitals was 'as good as can be obtained anywhere and that no criticism other than commendation can possibly be called for'.[144] Ball and Myles argued that some of the approved hospitals lacked surgical specialists. In these instances, they explained, it was their duty to give such assistance when required. They finished the letter by clarifying:

> as we have to report to the War Office ... we rely on the courtesy of the staff of hospitals receiving wounded soldiers to give us facilities for occasionally visiting these soldier patients, of course only in the presence of those in professional charge of such patients if they so desire.[145]

Eager to resolve the issue, the hospital committee explained that there was a division among their members on the matter. Some committee members argued that the provisions of the War Office circular were 'necessary for the control and working of what may be called "unguaranteed" institutions and that the circular might be accepted'.[146] Other members of the committee believed that a circular articulating the right of the War Office to supervise, criticise and possibly supersede members of the hospital staff should not be accepted.[147]

While this dispute was unfolding, an incident involving Myles' occurred at the Longford County Infirmary that emphasised the conflict between the civilian medical profession and military medical representatives in Ireland. In January 1915, Dr. Mayne, surgeon at the Longford County Infirmary, refused to allow Myles to operate on a soldier brought to the institution. Mayne was unprepared to let anyone, aside from himself, operate on the soldier who was suffering from appendicitis.[148] Consequently, a row erupted between Mayne and Myles with Myles later reporting that he had never seen anything like it in his long career. Yet Mayne held firm and ultimately, refused Myles permission to work in the operating theatre with the soldier transported elsewhere. In a letter entitled 'Professional etiquette and the RAMC' published in the *Medical Press*, Mayne reiterated that he was prepared to admit the soldier that had been brought to the infirmary by Myles but would not let 'any man operate in the hospital without his consent'. The editor of the *Medical Press* supported Mayne's decision and accepted that while surgeons in county infirmaries regularly allowed others to use their operating theatres, it was entirely at the behest of the surgeon.[149] Following the incident, Lord Granard, Lord Lieutenant of Longford, Colonel in the Royal Irish Regiment and an acquaintance of Myles, placed considerable political pressure on the governors of the Longford infirmary to dismiss Mayne from his role in the dispensary. Mayne was subsequently fired.[150]

In an attempt to ease the rising friction between civilian hospital and military staff, Surgeon General Anderson conceded that 'the paragraph [in the circular], "they will operate themselves in cases in which they consider such a course desirable and will advise others engaged in operative work" was not intended to apply to hospitals that already had their own consulting staff'.[151] In practice, the consulting surgeons' interference was minimal for the remainder of the war and they only performed operations in agreement with the hospital authorities or the institutions' medical staff.

While the DDMS' efforts went some way to appeasing hospital medical staff, discontent soon arose between the War Office and hospital governors regarding other matters. In an attempt to cut costs, the War Office issued an Army Council Instruction relating to the grants made to domestic class A auxiliary hospitals on behalf of soldiers. It stated that the grant should not exceed the actual expenditure of a hospital on maintenance, and they introduced a maximum grant rate of 3*s.* per day. Maintenance was defined under three headings: medicines, provisions—surgical dressings and stimulants—and renewals of furniture and bedding. The grant was not to be used to cover other items, including salaries of nurses. Instead, the hospital was to meet these costs through other sources.[152] Ireland's hospital governors, appalled by potential cuts to their War Office income, gathered to discuss a solution. On 13 November 1916, the governors of the Meath Hospital informed the War Office that the minimum cost of each soldier to the hospital was at least 3*s.* 6*d.* per day and any reduction in payments to the hospital would have hampered the hospital's treatment of sick and wounded soldiers.[153] Similar responses from Ireland's other civilian hospitals encouraged the War Office to retain the status-quo regarding payments and in practice there was no cut in hospital maintenance fees. It was, however, a sign of impending changes to the RAMC casualty clearing process and the dangers of the hospitals' growing reliance on income associated with the treatment of soldiers.

## Specialist Hospitals

Another notable change in the casualty clearing process, was the RAMC's increasing reliance on specialist military hospitals. From December 1914 until the end of the war, the number of hospital beds in Britain for the treatment of soldiers increased from 40,000 to 364,133.[154] This increase was in part due to the establishment of various specialist hospitals, including wards in district lunatic asylums for the treatment of soldiers suffering from mental difficulties.[155] Ben Shepherd has estimated that approximately seven per cent of British Army Officers and three per cent of other ranks suffered nervous and mental shock within the first three months of war.[156] From 1914 until the end of 1915, most soldiers suffering from shell-shock and diseases of the mind were returned to Britain for treatment.[157] Consequently, the RAMC's initial allocation of 1800 beds for shell-shock cases was inadequate and the corps required additional facilities to admit sufferers.[158] In 1915, the War Office requested the Board of Control for Lunacy and Mental Deficiency, which presided over all county and borough lunatic asylums in England and Wales, to provide 50,000 beds for soldiers.[159]

In the same year, the War Office granted William Dawson, Inspector of Lunatic Asylums in Ireland, the temporary rank of Lieutenant Colonel and appointed him as the specialist in nerve diseases for troops in Ireland. Dawson had considerable experience in dealing with patients suffering from mental illness. Previously, he had held posts at Farnham House, Dublin and Maryville Private Hospital for Mental Disease in Finglas, Dublin, and in 1911 he was appointed Inspector of Lunatic Asylums in Ireland. He had also been the President of the Irish division of the Medico-Psychological Association of Great Britain and Ireland prior to the outbreak of conflict.[160] Dawson was tasked with finding suitable accommodation in Ireland for the treatment of soldiers suffering from nerve diseases, a difficult assignment due to the overcrowded state of Irish asylums during this period.[161] Despite several expansion programmes carried out throughout the nineteenth century, Ireland's asylums were regularly overcrowded.[162] Prior to Dawson's appointment, soldiers with mental illness were housed in Ireland's general military hospitals, an arrangement which he recognised as 'never very satisfactory'.[163]

On 16 June 1916, Dawson took charge of a building located in Grangegorman Asylum in Dublin. Opened in 1815, Grangegorman Asylum, originally known as the Richmond Lunatic Asylum, was state-funded and admitted patients from its catchment area, which included the city and county of Dublin, the counties of Louth, Meath, Wicklow and the town of Drogheda.[164] The Grangegorman governors offered the War Office a building that could cater for thirty-two patients including soldiers domiciled in Dublin or those awaiting transfer to other institutions. Joseph Reynolds and Peter Reid have argued that the governors of the asylum opened the ward for soldiers to secure the War Office payment of 21s. per week, per occupied bed.[165] In his 1917 annual report, Dr. John Donelan, Resident Medical Superintendent of the asylum, recorded that wartime inflation had increased the cost of clothing, drugs and fuel by 'two to three hundred per cent' since 1913.[166] The War Office payment was thus attractive to the asylum's Governors.

From the date of opening in June 1916 until its closure on 23 December 1919, the Richmond War Hospital treated 362 cases, of which two-thirds were discharged to friends or general military hospitals; only two returned to duty and thirty-one were sent directly to civil asylums.[167] As the cost of the soldier's treatment was covered by the military, the RAMC supervised the asylum's war ward. On 1 August 1916, Lieutenant Colonel Hearn, an RAMC officer at King George V Hospital Dublin, informed Donelan that

> all soldier patients transferred to Richmond Asylum War Hospital remain under the control of the War Office and as officer in charge of King George V Hospital I am responsible for them no matter in what part of your asylum they may have to be accommodated until such time as they are invalided from the army.[168]

In 1917, despite the creation of special psychiatric treatment centres in France, the RAMC endeavoured to further increase accommodation for sufferers in Ireland and requested Dawson place a larger asylum of about 500 beds at the military's disposal.[169] Similar arrangements had been successfully introduced in Britain and the RAMC were in control of a number of asylums throughout the United Kingdom.[170] In April, following Dawson's recommendation, the War Office acquired Belfast's

Civil Lunatic Asylum and incorporated it into the Belfast War Hospital. At this time, the majority of Belfast asylum's patients were housed in a new facility in Purdysburn. However, there were still approximately 400 patients housed in the old building. Dawson and his colleagues decided that the only way to facilitate the War Office's request was to vacate the old asylum and rehouse the 400 or so civilian patients in other institutions. Most of the 400 were transferred to a separate department in the Belfast Union workhouse. While Dawson acknowledged that the situation was far from ideal, the transfer of psychiatric patients to the local workhouse was a relatively common practice in Ireland and was therefore seen as a solution to a difficult situation.[171]

Once the old Belfast asylum building was emptied, military patients— Irish men and those belonging to Irish regiments but not of Irish birth—arrived and increased the number of soldiers in Ireland requiring treatment for mental illness. The first cases arrived on 15 May 1917. Initially, the asylum staff remained to treat the soldiers; Dr. William Graham, Medical Superintendent of the Belfast Asylum, was central to the management of the institution during the soldiers' residence. Graham, who the RAMC had granted the temporary rank of Lieutenant Colonel, was an advocate of the 'virtues of open air, activities offered by agricultural labour, and of strict temperance' in the treatment of patients and it is probable that these methods were in place during his time in charge of military patients.[172] Graham's role at the Belfast institution was cut short due to his sudden death in November 1917, just seven months after the arrival of soldiers. Following Graham's passing, Dawson and the RAMC agreed that the corps would take full control of the asylum and assigned RAMC staff to manage the institution.[173] In December 1917, Lieutenant Colonel John P. J. Murphy, a County Cork native, took charge of the institution.[174] Between 1917 and the asylum's closure 1193 cases were admitted—772 were discharged into the care of their family or friends and the remainder transferred to other hospitals.[175]

During the war, the RAMC and voluntary groups also established several specialised orthopaedic hospitals in Britain and Ireland. Cooter has suggested that approximately sixty-five per cent of First World War casualties suffered injuries to locomotor functions due to damage caused by bullets and shells. Shrapnel and gunfire caused numerous injuries to legs, arms and various other parts of soldiers' bodies.[176] Public and medical interest in orthopaedics increased because of the First World War and it was no longer the 'butt of medical jokes'.[177] By 1918, there were twenty specialised orthopaedic hospitals in several locations throughout Britain, including Queen Mary's Auxiliary Hospital for Limbless Men at Roehampton, London, one of the most important orthopaedic institutions in Britain, which fitted tens of thousands of soldiers with artificial limbs during the war years.[178] The majority of Irish soldiers participants who suffered from locomotor injuries received treatment in Roehampton during the initial stages of the war.[179]

In 1915 the Red Cross and the SJA took over the Princess Patricia Hospital, Bray, County Wicklow, and approximately 180 men were treated there for injuries to locomotor functions. Richard Ford, who the RAMC had appointed as the Deputy Director of Medical Services, Irish Command in 1916, encouraged the Red Cross to further increase specialist facilities for orthopaedic cases and limbless soldiers. Consequently, in December 1916, a committee, comprising of several notable Irish philanthropists, including Viscountess Powerscourt; Sir Algernon, a member of the Guinness family and acting Lieutenant Commander in the Royal Naval Volunteer Reserve; and James Gallagher, Lord Mayor of Dublin, met in the Shelbourne Hotel, Dublin, to discuss the possibility of establishing a specialised facility for the treatment of limbless men in Ireland. Prior to the meeting, Ford had secured the support of several patrons for the hospital, including the Duke of Connaught, who gave his name to the institution.[180] The committee passed a number of resolutions during the initial meeting and outlined their aims:

> to establish a hospital for the care and treatment of Irish sailors and soldiers who have lost their limbs in this war while their artificial limbs are being fitted, and to give them such instruction as is possible while in hospital. And further, to do everything possible to promote the future welfare of these men after their discharge from hospital.[181]

On 12 December 1916, the Committee of the Duke of Connaught's Auxiliary Hospital for Irish Sailors and Soldiers launched an official public appeal for funds to allow them to acquire the Meath Industrial School for Girls, Bray, County Wicklow, and establish a hospital for the treatment of limbless soldiers on the site.[182] The committee reached an agreement with governors of the Meath Industrial School that, should the funds be raised, the committee would pay rent of £300 per annum for the period of the war and for one or two years afterwards. The committee members had identified the school as the ideal location for the hospital because of the spacious rooms that were large enough to accommodate workshops. The hospital would follow the example of similar institutions in France by providing workshops that would teach limbless soldiers 'tailoring, boot-making, carpentry and so on, with factories and showrooms ... to keep the men occupied'.[183]

Following large donations from the British Red Cross and SJA, the committee acquired the school and opened the hospital. The institution catered for approximately fifty limbless sailors and soldiers of Irish birth.[184] Further finance was raised shortly afterwards and the number of beds in the hospital rose to sixty. The two wards within the hospital—Guinness Ward and Holden Stodart Ward—were named in honour of the Guinness family, one of the hospital's largest donors, and Holden Stodart, a Guinness employee and a member of the SJA who had died after being shot while tending to the wounded during the Easter Rising.[185]

In late 1916, following major battles on the Western Front, including the Battle of the Somme, new facilities opened in Ireland for orthopaedic cases. In February 1917, the governors of the Ulster Volunteer Force Hospital in Belfast opened 236 new beds for the treatment of soldiers who had lost their limbs in the war and orthopaedic cases.[186] Lieutenant Colonel A. B. Mitchell, a fellow of the RCSI and member of the Royal Army Medical Corps, oversaw the ward and encouraged the construction of additional workshop rooms and a gymnasium. By April, approximately thirty-four limbless soldiers and 118 orthopaedic patients were in the hospital.[187] On 19 May 1917, the Blackrock Orthopaedic Hospital opened in Dublin under the control of Lieutenant Colonel T. J. Potter, a licentiate of the RCPI, who had commanded the 6th Field Ambulance in the early stages of the conflict. The War Office acquired the hospital buildings from the governors of the Meath Protestant Industrial Schools for Boys—the boys who had been in the school were moved to another industrial school in Belfast. Following the example of the Committee of the Duke of Connaught's Hospital and the UVF Hospital, Potter successfully sought substantial philanthropic support to fund the hospital and to equip it with beds for 520 patients. The main building consisted of eight wards but the majority of men were accommodated in huts in the grounds. Fifty-seven officers and 2453 men from other ranks were treated while 697 operations were performed and prosthetic limbs fitted.[188] Sir William Wheeler, renowned surgeon and TCD graduate, and Major Haughton, member of the RAMC, carried out the work at Blackrock and according to Ireland's Deputy Director of Medical

Services, the hospital was 'at least equal to any hospital of its kind in the United Kingdom'.[189]

Elsewhere in Ireland, the RAMC opened other wards and hospitals to accommodate for returned soldiers who suffered from contagious diseases. In May 1917, the RAMC classified the Curragh Military Hospital as the centre for the treatment of tubercular cases among soldiers. The Curragh Military Hospital, which was one of the oldest military hospitals in Ireland, was outdated and ill-prepared for the stresses placed upon it during the First World War. Due to the lack of appropriate space and facilities, doctors at the hospital had only treated the 'lighter class of cases' returning from the British Expeditionary Force prior to its classification as a hospital for treating tuberculosis sufferers.[190] Tuberculosis was prevalent among soldiers fighting in several regions, including France and the Eastern Front. Leo Van Bergen has calculated that almost the entire bed capacity of French tuberculosis clinics was reserved for soldiers and the disease was an everyday problem for most armies involved in the conflict.[191] Prior to the war, Ireland had one of the highest tuberculosis mortality rates in Europe. These rates increased during the conflict.[192]

The Curragh Military Hospital was strongly criticised by the Deputy Director of Medical Services who stated that it was in need of 'considerable improvement'.[193] The RAMC housed military patients in two wooden huts attached to the hospital and soldiers treated there criticised it publicly. One anonymous combatant wrote to the *Kildare Observer*:

> to enlighten the public the treatment the wounded soldier receives in this hospital. The food is disgraceful for wounded men returning from France. The dinner is worse that troops receive in barrack rooms or trenches. Smoking is strictly prohibited. No cigarettes are issued, and nobody is allowed to have money in their possession. This is not a frivolous complaint as you will see for yourself if you come to this "Prison". Hoping you will oblige.[194]

The editor of the *Observer* appended a response to the letter:

> We publish the letter in the hope that if the complaints are justified they will be seen without delay. This is the least concession due to the soldiers' home suffering from wounds honourably received in the performance of strenuous duty. It is highly indesirable [sic] from every point of view that they should have anything to complain of that can be remedied.[195]

The lack of alternative military medical facilities and civilian tuberculosis hospitals in Ireland, coupled with the small number of tuberculosis sufferers returned to Ireland—approximately 508 cases—ensured that the Curragh Military Hospital remained an important treatment centre despite being unsuitable.[196] Yet to provide additional support to the Curragh, the RAMC also arranged for civilian sanatoria to treat soldiers. By 1915, the Newcastle Hospital for Consumptives, located in County Wicklow, had reserved approximately twenty-five of its 135 beds for military personnel.[197]

The Curragh Military Hospital also became a specialist institution for the treatment of malaria cases. Malaria inflicted more casualties in the British Army than any other disease in its history of overseas campaigns.[198] The British Army's extension into Salonika, East Africa and the Middle East from 1915 onwards brought troops into contact with the disease. Approximately 34,000 soldiers suffering from severe and obstinate cases returned to Britain for treatment.[199] The RAMC chose the Curragh as the treatment site in Ireland and again the hospital lacked the appropriate facilities. Cases had to be accommodated on the general medical wards but the RAMC continued to use the hospital to house malaria patients because of the relatively small number of sufferers returned to Ireland.[200]

Outbreaks of venereal diseases (VD) prompted a more committed response from the RAMC in Ireland.[201] Whitehead has estimated that sufferers of VD numbered approximately 287 per 1000 among some British regiments.[202] Several initiatives were introduced by the War Office to halt the spread of VD, including the stoppage of pay for any soldier admitted to hospital suffering from the disease; yet it remained a significant problem. Due to the rising number of sufferers in Britain, political interest in combating VD increased. In 1916, the Royal Commission on Venereal Diseases recommended that local authorities should establish clinics providing free and anonymous treatment and central government should contribute seventy-five per cent of the cost.[203] According to Susannah Riordan, these new recommendations were implemented in England, Wales and Scotland with speed and efficiency, but not in Ireland. As a result of the disarray in the system of local government during the period of political unrest, there was a significant legislative delay which prevented the introduction of the recommendations.[204]

The rapid increase in the number of VD cases among military men emphasised the inadequacy of pre-existing facilities for their treatment in Ireland. Initially, soldiers suffering from VD were treated in the Military Hospital, Portobello in Dublin, which had approximately 100 beds. Irish civilian hospital governors were reluctant to accept venereal patients into their institutions and in April 1918, the RAMC opened a new special-ised VD hospital at Fort Westmoreland, on Spike Island off the coast of County Cork.[205] There was a considerable amount of local protest to the opening of the facility.[206] At a conference of the Bishop of Cork and the priests of Cork City, those present objected to the establish-ment of the hospital.[207] In March 1918, J. Lane, a member of the Cork Union Board of Guardians, requested that the Irish population oppose the establishment of venereal hospitals in the country, and that 'all for-eigners so suffering be immediately deported to their own country'.[208] However, the hospital was established and by 1919, it accommodated approximately 600 military patients.[209]

The outbreak of the First World War thus prompted an expansion of specialist military hospitals throughout Ireland. Facilities were estab-lished in direct response to injuries and diseases that were prominent among soldiers. Given the increasing move towards specialist hospital provision, it is necessary to explore the impact the opening these institu-tions had on civilian hospitals and the role they played in the treatment of soldiers for the remainder of the war.

## CIVILIAN HOSPITALS, 1917–1918

Harrison has posited that by mid-1916, the RAMC treated more sol-diers closer to the front rather than transport them home as it was both cheaper and more effective.[210] Yet there was little immediate evi-dence of this in Ireland.[211] More sick and wounded soldiers were trans-ported to Ireland in 1917 than at any other point in the war.[212] From the beginning of June until the end of July 1917, ships of wounded soldiers arrived in Ireland on a near weekly basis. It was not until the winter months that the number of soldiers returned to Ireland began to slow down before really dwindling in 1918. Due to the increase in spe-cialist military facilities and proposed changes to the casualty dispersal plan, the RAMC sought to reduce the number of beds reserved for sol-diers in Ireland's civilian hospitals. On 21 September 1917, Lieutenant

Colonel Thomas Clarke, RAMC, contacted the governors of the House of Industry Hospitals:

> I am directed to inform you that with the approach of winter, it is felt by the military authorities that they should relinquish their claims on 40 beds in your hospital … in order to release more beds for the needs of the civil community, more especially as we are not now receiving many sick and wounded from overseas. At the same time, we should like to feel if necessity should again arise for more accommodation, that we could count on our original number of beds provided that we gave you adequate notice, as the Military Authorities highly appreciate the care, skill, and attention with which our wounded and sick soldiers have been treated in your institution.[213]

On 7 December, Richard Ford reiterated to the hospital governors that it was unlikely the beds reserved for soldiers in the hospitals would be utilised.[214] Yet, the governors continued to reserve beds for soldiers, even though they were empty.[215] It is likely that this was a result of an agreement they had reached with the War Office earlier in the year that guaranteed 6*d.* per day for each unoccupied bed.[216]

While this was a modest amount, it was an additional income stream at a time when the financial problems continued to adversely effect on civilian hospitals. On 31 March 1917, the Secretary of the House of Industry Hospitals reported that 'as prices steadily increased more, especially in the last three months … it is quite apparent that the year we have just entered into will be an even worse one financially than its predecessor'.[217] Hospitals' debt continued to mount. In December 1917, the governors of Sir Patrick Dun's Hospital reported a considerable debt of £6352.[218] In an attempt to improve the financial position of the hospital, the governors examined the possibility of implementing a cost-cutting measure of closing some beds open to civilians. In a public statement, issued as part of the hospital's annual report, the governors explained that 'owing to the very large increase in the cost of food and of surgical and medical appliances, etc. it is most difficult to keep open all the beds. They now look more than ever to the public for the necessary funds to pay current expenses'.[219] Before the war, similar public appeals had been successful in raising funds and it was predictable that the governors adopted a similar tactic during the concluding stages of the war, which were especially financially difficult. The public response, however, was less than enthusiastic. Hospital income from subscriptions and bequests declined in 1918.[220] The Royal City of Dublin Hospital governors also registered a decrease in donations, bemoaning that 'alas, not all our friends are immune from the great financial struggle for existence brought about by war. As a natural consequence, many of our annual contributions have been considerably reduced and some have been discontinued'.[221]

It is possible that changes in public attitudes towards war were partly responsible for the decline in public donations to some of the hospitals. Republican organisations multiplied throughout Ireland in the final two years of the war and, as this wave of separatist nationalism increased, hostility was directed towards the British Army and those serving in it.[222] Some separatists questioned whether the Irish population should continue funding the treatment of British Army soldiers, particularly when fellow nationalist insurgents had suffered injury in domestic conflict and required medical treatment. In 1917, a member of Cumann na MBan, an Irish republican women's paramilitary organisation formed in Dublin in 1914, complained in *Nationality*, a nationalist publication edited by Arthur Griffith, that 'there are Irish men and women devoting all their time and attention to English Wounded soldiers, and are we going to neglect our own'?.[223] Similar attitudes may have had a negative impact on the civilian hospitals' ability to raise funds through donations and subscriptions.

Yet it is more likely that the sheer number of fundraising efforts in Ireland for the benefit of sick and wounded soldiers in the latter years of the war diverted direct subscriptions away from the hospitals. In 1917 and 1918, for instance, the Joint War Committee of the British Red Cross Society and St. John's Ambulance Brigade in Leinster, Munster and Connaught established a committee of management to organise a more coordinated drive for charitable donations to fund their wartime activities. Sir John Arnott, chairman of the *Irish Times*, strongly supported the committee and advertised initiatives such as 'Our Day' freely in the newspaper, while the Lord Lieutenant chaired a public meeting in the Royal Dublin Society lecture theatre to raise awareness. The committee of management, county directors and those involved organised flag days, concerts, sports events and church collections as part of the drive and £132,000 was raised across the two years (£62,000 in 1917 and £70,000 in 1918).[224] Approximately £64,000 of this total was raised in Dublin. Due to the financial difficulties brought on by war, the public could only support so many fundraising efforts with high-profile initiatives such as 'Our Day' prospering and consequently, hospital subscription rates fell.

In Ulster, the Royal Victoria Hospital in Belfast, who largely garnered its funds from the unionist community, was one of the few Irish hospitals that reported a profit during the final two years of war and this was largely due to its connections with local industry.[225] In a 1916 appeal for funds, Lady Pirrie, President of the Hospital, encouraged potential subscribers to recognise that 'the Royal Victoria Hospital bore the name of the illustrious Sovereign whose reign was unique in British history ... it was thus associated with the ideals of British Royalty and Imperial progress'.[226] While the hospital's debt had rapidly accumulated between 1914 and 1916, it's income increased considerably in 1917.[227] Reflecting on the hospital's financial year in 1917, Sir William Crawford, chairman of the hospital's board of management, noted that the hospital's expenditure had doubled to £30,000 when compared to figures in pre-war years. However, due to 'a few men who did not wish to have their efforts made public, their [the hospital's] funds were in a better position than when they were spending the smaller sum'.[228] During this period, the political, social and commercial unionist elite, who were heavily involved in the hospital, utilised their connections in local business to organise successful workplace collections from employees throughout Belfast including those in railway companies and local shipyards such as Harland and Wolff.[229] Income from subscriptions and other events soon soared to record levels.[230]

While the financial support for the Royal Victoria Hospital went largely against the trends evident in hospital accounts elsewhere in Ireland, the institution, like other hospitals, was still dependent on the War Office's payments. In its 1918 press release, the hospital's Saturday Committee, a fundraising group, emphasised that the Royal Victoria Hospital's total annual income of £31,729 included £3536, which was received by the War Office for the maintenance of wounded soldiers and

had it not been for this, the balance of the bank would have been on the wrong side of the account. When the war was over, the beds would no longer be required by the military, the money they now received for them would be stopped and this would have to be made good in some way or other, because the expenses would go on just the same as the beds vacated by soldiers would be required.[231]

Thus, despite its profitable subscriber list, the Royal Victoria Hospital in Belfast was, like other hospitals in Ireland, in a financially perilous position in the final years of the conflict.

## CIVILIAN PATIENTS

Given the financial difficulties faced by the civilian hospitals and the coinciding influx of soldiers into their wards for the duration of war, it is appropriate to explore the impact of the conflict on the management of civilian patients in the hospitals. Abel-Smith has suggested that the departure of a significant number of doctors to participate in the First World War eroded the standards of care for the civilian sick in hospitals.[232] There is no doubt that hospitals in Ireland lost experienced medical staff for the duration of the war. Hospital governors had demonstrated concern about staffing levels since the beginning of the conflict when members of the medical staff started to enlist. In their 1914 annual report, governors of Sir Patrick Dun's Hospital had claimed that seventeen nurses had volunteered for service and the 'nursing staff was somewhat diminished'.[233] The concerns of governors intensified as the war progressed and staff shortages became more severe. By May 1917, for example, seven out of ten members of the Royal City of Dublin Hospital regular medical staff were away on war service.[234]

However, neither newspaper or journal articles, nor hospital records and inspection board reports, reveal specific evidence of a decline in the standard of civilian healthcare due to staff shortages. Wartime reports from the Board of Superintendence of Dublin Hospitals explicitly note that staff shortages did not affect civilian healthcare in the hospitals they examined. In 1918, the board reported that while several staff at the Richmond, Whitworth and Hardwicke Hospitals were serving in the army, they found 'work being carried on very much as usual, owing to the remaining staff taking on increased duties'.[235] Likewise, following an inspection of the Meath Hospital, the board claimed that 'with a staff diminished by the call of war, [the hospital] does its work as usual. After a very critical inspection we have nothing but good to say of it'.[236] It is important to note here that while the Board of Superintendence of Dublin Hospitals' reports provide an intriguing insight into the workings of Dublin hospitals, they cannot be relied on to wholly provide an impartial viewpoint on the workings of the hospitals. The board had a membership of twelve and among them were representatives of the boards of managements of the hospitals being inspected and they were thus were unlikely to be critical of their own institutions.[237]

Yet, their opinions cannot be totally discounted. Hospital governors were able to somewhat offset the loss of doctors and nurses to war using three different methods. Firstly, they hired additional staff, usually junior medical personnel, when staffing levels were low during the war. Unlike poor law dispensaries, hospital governors could hire young doctors. In their 1916 annual report, the medical staff of the Royal Victoria Hospital in Belfast thanked several doctors, including Dr. Coates; Dr. Elwood and Dr. Taggart, who had 'filled to a very large extent the places of the members of the regular staff who were absent on war service'.[238] Most of the replacements were eligible to serve in the war.[239] Secondly, hospitals utilised their long-standing relationships with local medical schools and medical students took increasing responsibility for medical care on the wards during the war. On 19 March 1915, for instance, governors of the House of Industry Hospitals granted a request from their medical staff to appoint additional junior physicians and surgeons to try and assist remaining staff 'owing to the amount of work … through the absence of some of the staff serving in the war'.[240] In the same month, a fifth-year student qualified in surgery was appointed as junior and house surgeon for six months without salary, but he was provided with free board and lodging.[241] Similarly, the medical staff of the Royal Victoria Hospital, Belfast, noted that because of 'the shortage of qualified residents' the governors had decided that fifth year students would act as resident clinical assistants at a salary of £30 per annum.[242] Finally, when governors believed that there was a danger of losing all experienced staff, they stopped granting leave to those requesting to go to war. This was particularly evident in 1918. On 12 April 1918, for instance, the Royal City of Dublin Hospital governors refused a request from George Johnston for a further 3 months leave of absence to continue his duties as Lieutenant Colonel in the RAMC.[243] Through prudent staff management, governors were thus able to alleviate the effect of wartime staff shortages on the standard of healthcare in Irish hospitals.

This is not to say that civilian healthcare was unaffected by war but rather, the conflict negatively affected civilians in Irish hospitals in several other ways. In response to the financial crisis brought on by war, many of the hospitals that admitted paying patients increased their prices. In June 1918, the Royal Victoria Eye and Ear Hospital, Dublin, increased its charges from 3s. to 4s. per day, as hospital authorities believed that they had 'no alternative due to rising prices and falling off in subscriptions owing to war'.[244] Likewise, the Incorporated Orthopaedic Hospital, Dublin, announced that the charges made as 'contribution in aid' for maintenance of patients in the hospital had increased from a rate of 12s. per week for children and 15s. for adults to a flat rate of 18s. per head, per week.[245] Financial difficulties brought on by war thus increased the cost of medical care for civilians in Ireland.

Civilians' access to hospital care was also hindered due to the admission of soldiers to the wards. While several hospitals, including Sir Patrick Dun's, underwent construction that resulted in the creation of new wards for soldiers, others admitted military patients into wards previously reserved for civilians and this limited the accommodation available. As early as February 1915, Sir Charles Ball claimed that all the clinical hospitals in Belfast, Cork and Dublin had 'thrown open their wards [for soldiers], but this had prevented them from giving necessary attention to ordinary civilian cases'.[246] At the 1916 annual meeting of the supporters of the Adelaide Hospital, Dublin, the secretary announced that 472 patients had been admitted to the medical wards of the hospital in 1915; a figure well below the average number of admissions. The Adelaide Committee acknowledged that 'the decrease was accounted for by the fact that Victoria House [a medical ward] was still occupied by wounded soldiers. This during the year has caused considerable inconvenience, as the staff had to refuse all [civilian] infectious cases which were sent for admission to the hospital'.[247] Hospital authorities were thus turning civilian patients away in favour of military cases.

To ensure that public donations to Dublin hospitals were not affected in 1917, the Committee of the Dublin Hospital Sunday Fund released a statement to counteract public opposition to the hospitals' admittance of soldiers ahead of civilians: 'it was objected in some quarters that soldiers were taking the places that ought to be available in the hospitals for civilians, but the truth was the soldiers were not interfering materially with the treatment of civilians'.[248] Despite these denials, hospital authorities' prioritisation of military cases was evident for the remainder of the war. In November 1917, for instance, the medical staff of the House of Industry Hospitals inquired of the governors whether civilians could be admitted to the soldiers' ward when the other wards were crowded. The governors granted permission but on the condition that the ward 'be immediately be given up for military patients when required'.[249]

Similarly, the influx of military patients into the Belfast Asylum in 1917 pushed 400 civilian patients out of the asylum and into the workhouse. While the process of moving the patients elsewhere was already in train, the impending arrival of soldiers forced the authorities to reach a quick resolution and patients were transferred into an institution not designed to accommodate them. This was not an isolated incident. Since 1915, several boards of guardians had complained about the influx of cases into the workhouse due to the presence of soldiers in local hospitals. In May 1915, the North Dublin Union Board of Guardians had complained that due to the soldiers' presence in hospitals, the citizens were pushed into the workhouse and 'deprived of the accommodation they ought to get'.[250] War thus limited civilian access to hospital care in Ireland and encouraged their admission to workhouse facilities.

Civilian healthcare was also affected by a scarcity of drugs that were difficult to secure, as supplies were limited due to conflict. In their 1916 annual report, the LGBI noted that they had been hampered when preparing their annual drug list because 'many important drugs in general use for some years past had become very scarce and expensive'.[251] For instance, the price of Potassii Bromidum, Sodii Bromidum and Sodii Salicylas had increased significantly, from 2s. and 3d., 2s. and 9d., and 2s. a pound, respectively, to 30s., 24s. and 25s. a pound.[252] While the effectiveness of many of these drugs was limited, the rising prices encouraged the LGBI to stop buying drugs which either were 'unprocurable or had reached a prohibitive figure'.[253] Given the rising expenditure on drugs in hospitals, it is unlikely that hospitals stopped buying medicines but rather medical staff became economic when prescribing. A similar strategy was in practice in the poor law dispensaries. On 12 March 1918, J. E. Devlin, Assistant Secretary of the LGBI, informed several boards of guardians that due to conflict, the 'dearth of drugs [was] daily becoming more marked and medical officers are strongly urged to restrict their demands on the general supplies to the smallest amounts'.[254]

## CONCLUSION

This chapter has identified that military hospitals constituted a much larger percentage of the total accommodation for soldiers in Ireland than in Britain during the war because of local Irish conditions, namely, the unsuitability of Irish infrastructure. Yet Ireland's civilian hospitals were also central to the provision of beds for soldiers. While institutional histories have tended to focus on the positive contribution of hospital staff to the treatment of soldiers, this chapter posits that ultimately Ireland's hospitals suffered during the war. The rising levels of wartime inflation offset the financial benefits received from treating soldiers.

In addition, this chapter suggests that Ireland's hospital governors largely managed staff levels well throughout the war and utilising their relationships with local universities, brought in additional junior medical staff as required. This went someway to alleviating the ill effects the war had on civilian medical care but ultimately the war had a negative bearing on the provision of hospital care for civilians in Ireland. Soldiers occupied beds in civilian hospitals, pushing civilians into institutions not designed to treat them. Rising inflation, and problems with supplies, also increased the cost of hospital care for paying patients.

## NOTES

1. Report of Deputy Director of Medical Services, Irish Command, 26 January 1920 (TNA, Irish situation, 1914–1922 collection, WO 35 179).
2. Harrison, *The medical war*, p. 17.
3. Harrison, *The medical war*, pp. 1–15.
4. Van Bergen has examined military hospitals in the Netherlands in the First World War and argued that of the 44 military hospitals in the Netherlands, only 12 were originally intended for medical use and many were unsuitable and in urgent need of renovation. For more, see Leo Van Bergen, "'The malingerers are to blame': The Dutch military health service before and during the First World War" in Cooter et al. (eds.), *Medicine and modern warfare*, p. 67.
5. MacPherson, *History of the Great War*, p. 71.
6. Report of Deputy Director of Medical Services, Irish Command, 26 January 1920 (TNA, Irish situation, 1914–1922 collection, WO 35 179).
7. Report of Deputy Director of Medical Services, Irish Command, 26 January 1920 (TNA, Irish situation, 1914–1922 collection, WO 35 179); This figure is based on calculating the number of hospitals ships and the average number of wounded contained on each as per the DDMS report. However, it is most likely an underestimation. The report does not contain a record of all hospital ships docked in Ireland. It is also important to note that this figure does not indicate the total number of wounded soldiers that received treatment in Ireland during the war

as not all wounded returned on hospital ships. Some soldiers returned to Ireland by other transport and were subsequently admitted by the RAMC into the hospitals. Also see, *The Red Cross in Ireland*, p. 26.

8. Report of Deputy Director of Medical Services, Irish Command, 26 January 1920 (TNA, Irish situation, 1914–1922 collection, WO 35 179).

9. See Appendix: Tables B5 and C1.

10. Laurence Geary, *Medicine and charity in Ireland, 1718–1851* (Dublin: University College Dublin Press, 2004), p. 2.

11. Helen Burke, *The Royal Hospital, Donnybrook: A heritage of caring, 1743–1993* (Dublin: Royal Hospital Donnybrook and the Social Science Research Centre, 1993); Davis Coakley, *Baggot Street: A short history of the Royal City of Dublin Hospital* (Dublin: Board of Governors, Royal City of Dublin Hospital, 1995); Davis Coakley, *Doctor Steevens' Hospital* (Dublin: Dr. Steevens' Hospital Historical Centre, 1992); E.T. Freeman, *Mater Misericordiae Hospital: Centenary, 1861–1961* (Dublin, 1962); Peter Gatenby, *Dublin's Meath Hospital, 1753–1996* (Dublin: Town House, 1996); T.P.C. Kirkpatrick, *History of Dr Steevens' Hospital, Dublin, 1720–1920* (Dublin: University Press, 1924); F.O.C. Meenan (ed.), *The Children's Hospital, Temple Street, Dublin, 1872–1972* (Dublin, 1972); David Mitchell, *'A peculiar place': The Adelaide Hospital, Dublin, 1839–1989* (Dublin, 1989); T.G. Moorhead, *A short history of Sir Patrick Dun's Hospital* (Dublin: Hodges, Figgis, 1942); Joseph Reynolds, *Grangegorman: Psychiatric care in Dublin since 1815* (Dublin: Institute of Public Administration, 1992), J.D.H. Widdess, *The Charitable Infirmary, Jervis Street, 1718–1968* (Dublin, 1968); J.D.H. Widdess, *The Richmond, Whitworth and Hardwicke hospitals, St Laurence's Dublin, 1772–1972* (Dublin, 1972).

12. Winter, *The Great War*, pp. 154–172.

13. Harrison, *The medical war*, p. 65.

14. Anon., 'Hospital ships for the Tigris' in *British Medical Journal*, 2946, no. 1 (1917), p. 819.

15. See Appendix C: Table C2.

16. *Irish Times*, 31 October 1914; 'Hospital Ship, 1910–1929', ON 311 A, British Pathé.

17. For more on hospital design, see Jonathan Hughes, '"The matchbox on a muffin": The design of hospitals in the early NHS' in *Medical History*, 44, no. 1 (2000), pp. 21–56; Annmarie Adams, *Medicine by design: The architect and the modern hospital, 1893–1943* (Minnesota: University of Minnesota Press, 2008).

18. *Irish Times*, 19 September 1914.

19. Harrison, *The medical war*, p. 59.

20. *Irish Times*, 19 September 1914.
21. *The Red Cross in Ireland*, p. 27.
22. *Irish Times*, 1 September 1914.
23. *Irish Times*, 31 October 1914. Other newspapers published similar reports, including *Evening Herald*, 26 October 1914; *Fermanagh Herald*, 14 November 1914; *Irish Examiner*, 6 November 1914.
24. *Irish Times*, 31 October 1914.
25. *Irish Times*, 14 November 1914.
26. *Irish Times*, 4 September 1944. Within three months of the outbreak of the conflict, Lumsden had also established three auxiliary hospitals at Temple Hill, Blackrock; Monkstown and Mountjoy Square and used his own residence as a clearing house.
27. Order of St. John, *The Red Cross in Ireland*, p. 41.
28. For more, see Patrick Maume, 'Gordon (Marjoribanks), Dame Ishbel Maria marchioness of Aberdeen and Temair' in McGuire and Quinn (eds.), *Dictionary of Irish Biography*, iv, 141.
29. *Sinn Féin* was a weekly Irish nationalist newspaper, published from 1906 to 1914, edited by the founder of *Sinn Féin* party Arthur Griffith. The *Irish Worker* was a weekly publication, printed from May 1911 to December 1914, edited by James Larkin. Larkin was a trade union leader and founded the Irish Transport and General Workers' Union and the Irish Labour Party. He was a significant figure in the 1913 Dublin Lockout. See Emmet O'Connor, 'Larkin, James' in McGuire and Quinn (eds.), *Dictionary of Irish Biography*, v, 318; For more on both publications, see James Carty, *Bibliography of Irish History, 1912–21* (Dublin, 1936).
30. Letter from Lady Aberdeen to the editor of the *Freeman's Journal*, published in the *Irish Times*, 31 October 1914.
31. Letter from Denis Pack-Beresford to Lady Aberdeen, published in the *Irish Times*, 31 October 1914.
32. Letter from Lady Aberdeen to Denis Pack-Beresford, published in the *Irish Times*, 31 October 1914.
33. Order of St. John, *The Red Cross in Ireland*, p. 25.
34. Royal Irish Automobile Club, *War services presented to S. P. Anderson as a record of assistance given in connection with the wounded soldier's reception committee* (Dublin: Royal Irish Automobile Club, 1919).
35. Order of St. John, *The Red Cross in Ireland*, p. 25.
36. Report of Deputy Director of Medical Services, Irish Command, 26 January 1920 (TNA, Irish situation, 1914–1922 collection, WO 35 179).
37. For more on Dublin's medical infrastructure, see Mary E. Daly, *Dublin the deposed capital: A social and economic history, 1860–1914* (Cork: Cork University Press, 1984); Mary E. Daly, 'A tale of two cities:

1860–1920' in Art Cosgrove (ed.), *Dublin through the ages* (Dublin: College Press, 1988), pp. 113–131.

38. Abel-Smith, *The hospitals*, p. 253.
39. Abel-Smith, *The hospitals*, p. 253.
40. MacPherson, *History of the Great War*, p. 94.
41. Report of Deputy Director of Medical Services, Irish Command, 26 January 1920 (TNA, Irish situation, 1914–1922 collection, WO 35 179); Richard Ford replaced Russell as DDMS, Irish Command during the War.
42. Percentage based on calculations of the peak number of beds available in both military hospitals and other institutions treating soldiers taken from various figures and tables in the Report of Deputy Director of Medical Services, Irish Command, 26 January 1920 (TNA, Irish situation, 1914–1922 collection, WO 35 179).
43. Calculations based on figures contained in Report of Deputy Director of Medical Services, Irish Command, 26 January 1920 (TNA, Irish situation, 1914–1922 collection, WO 35 179).
44. Report of Deputy Director of Medical Services, Irish Command, 26 January 1920 (TNA, Irish situation, 1914–1922 collection, WO 35 179).
45. Other appointments included: Dr. Richard Matthews, surgeon at the Royal Victoria, Dr. Steevens' and Drumcondra hospitals; Dr. Herbert Mooney, ophthalmic surgeon at St. Vincent's and Temple Street hospitals; Dr. Thomas Graham, surgeon of the throat and nose at the Royal Victoria, Dublin and Royal City of Dublin hospitals; and Captain S.H.S. Taylor and Captain W.L. Murphy as eye, ear, nose and throat specialists. For more, see *Medical Directory*, 1914.
46. See Appendix B: Table B1.
47. *Irish Times*, 23 June 1917.
48. James Barrett, 'Trachoma and visual standards during the war' in *British Medical Journal*, 2953, no. 2 (1917), p. 97.
49. Report of Deputy Director of Medical Services, Irish Command, 26 January 1920 (TNA, Irish situation, 1914–1922 collection, WO 35 179).
50. Anon., 'Sir F. Conway Dwyer, M.D., F.R.C.S.I', *British Medical Journal*, 3902, no. 2 (1935), p. 765.
51. Report of Deputy Director of Medical Services, Irish Command, 26 January 1920 (TNA, Irish situation, 1914–1922 collection, WO 35 179).
52. Report of Deputy Director of Medical Services, Irish Command, 26 January 1920 (TNA, Irish situation, 1914–1922 collection, WO 35 179).
53. See Appendix: Table C2. The figures recorded by the DDMS for the year 1915 are incomplete. They only list three hospital ships arrivals

in Dublin from August onwards. However, a survey of the newspapers including the *Irish Times*, *Irish Examiner* and *Irish Independent* demonstrate that at least 6 docked that year.

54. Report of Deputy Director of Medical Services, Irish Command, 26 January 1920 (TNA, Irish situation, 1914–1922 collection, WO 35 179).
55. Harrison, *The medical war*, p. 65.
56. Report of Deputy Director of Medical Services, Irish Command, 26 January 1920 (TNA, Irish situation, 1914–1922 collection, WO 35 179).
57. *Donegal News*, 14 November 1914.
58. *Irish Times*, 16 November 1914.
59. *Belfast Newsletter*, 7 January 1915; *Irish Times*, 16 November 1914.
60. *Irish Times*, 16 November 1914; For more on Carson, see Alvin Jackson, 'Carson, Edward Henry Baron Carson of Duncairn' in McGuire and Quinn (eds.), *Dictionary of Irish Biography*, ii, 383.
61. *Irish Times*, 16 November 1914.
62. See Appendix B: Table B2.
63. James Craig was a prominent Irish unionist politician. He became the first Prime Minister of Northern Ireland. See Alvin Jackson, 'Craig, James 1st Viscount Craigavon' in McGuire and Quinn (eds.), *Dictionary of Irish Biography*, ii, 953; The Union Jack Committee, a unionist group, donated funds to the hospital. See *Irish Times*, 3 February 1909.
64. Report of Deputy Director of Medical Services, Irish Command, 26 January 1920 (TNA, Irish situation, 1914–1922 collection, WO 35 179).
65. See Appendix B: Table B3.
66. Report of Deputy Director of Medical Services, Irish Command, 26 January 1920 (TNA, Irish situation, 1914–1922 collection, WO 35 179).
67. See Appendix B: Table B4.
68. Report of Deputy Director of Medical Services, Irish Command, 26 January 1920 (TNA, Irish situation, 1914–1922 collection, WO 35 179).
69. Report of Deputy Director of Medical Services, Irish Command, 26 January 1920 (TNA, Irish situation, 1914–1922 collection, WO 35 179).
70. Report of Deputy Director of Medical Services, Irish Command, 26 January 1920 (TNA, Irish situation, 1914–1922 collection, WO 35 179).
71. 'Report of Assistant Director of Medical Services, 6th Division', 16 December 1919 (TNA, Irish situation, 1914–1922 collection, WO 35 179).
72. *Irish Times*, 30 November 1914.
73. *Irish Times*, 30 November 1914.
74. William Martin Murphy was a businessman and owner of the *Irish Independent* newspaper. He was a central figure in the Dublin employers' resistance to the Irish Transport and General Workers' Union, which ultimately led to the 1913 Lockout—when Murphy locked

out members of the ITGWU employed by the *Irish Independent*. He strongly supported Irish participation in the First World War. For more on Murphy, see Patrick Maume, 'Murphy, William Martin' in McGuire and Quinn (eds.), *Dictionary of Irish Biography*, vi, 825.

75. *Irish Times*, 30 November 1914.
76. *Irish Times*, 30 November 1914.
77. *Irish Times*, 30 November 1914.
78. Anon., 'Dublin Castle Hospital: Important statement and appeal for funds', p. 2.
79. Anon., 'Dublin Castle Hospital: Important statement and appeal for funds', p. 2.
80. Anon., 'Dublin Castle Hospital: Important statement and appeal for funds', p. 2.
81. *Is Dublin Castle suitable as a Red Cross Hospital: Report on Sanitary Conditions'* (NAI, Women's National Health Association papers, PRIV1212/WNHA/4/77).
82. Helen Andrews, 'Cameron, Sir Charles Alexander' in McGuire and Quinn (eds.), *Dictionary of Irish Biography*, ii, 271; For more on Cameron, see Lydia Carroll, *In the fever king's preserves: Sir Charles Cameron and the Dublin slums* (Dublin: A. & A. Farmar, 2011).
83. Anon., 'Dublin Castle Hospital: Important statement and appeal for funds', p. 2.
84. Anon., 'Dublin Castle Hospital: Important statement and appeal for funds', p. 2.
85. Lady Aberdeen formed the Women's National health Association of Ireland in 1907 to take part in the fight against tuberculosis. For more info on the association, see *Ulster Medical Journal* 1989; 58(Supplement): pp. 24–29; Minutes of Council Meetings of Women's National health Association of Ireland, December 1914 (NAI, Women's National Health Association papers, PRIV/1212/WNHA/1/3).
86. Dublin Castle Hospital minute book, 7 December 1914 (RCPI, Bound Manuscripts, BMS/5).
87. MacPherson, *History of the Great War*, p. 372.
88. Harrison, *The medical war*, p. 197.
89. Meath Hospital minute book, 31 August 1914 (NAI, 2007/128/5-3).
90. *Medical directory*, 1913, pp. 1541–1543.
91. Geary, *Medicine and charity in Ireland*, p. 2.
92. David Durnin, '"Medicine in the city": The impact of the National Insurance Act on health care and the medical profession in Dublin' in Mary Clark, Francis Devine, and Máire Kennedy (eds.), *A capital in conflict: Dublin City and the 1913 Lockout* (Dublin: Dublin City Council, 2013), pp. 83–106; Marie Coleman, *The Irish sweep: A history*

*of the Irish hospitals sweepstake, 1930–87* (Dublin: University College Dublin Press, 2009), pp. 1–22.

93. Meath Hospital minute book, 31 August 1914 (NAI, 2007/128/5-3).
94. Meath Hospital minute book, 31 August 1914 (NAI, 2007/128/5-3).
95. See Appendix B: Table B4 and Appendix C: Table C1.
96. Jay Winter, 'Hospitals' in Jay Winter and Jean-Louis Robert (eds.), *Capital cities at war: Paris, London, Berlin, 1914–19: A cultural history* (2 vols, Cambridge: Cambridge University Press, 2012), ii, 356.
97. See Appendix: Table B5.
98. For discussion of the financial crisis, see Durnin, 'Medicine in the city', pp. 83–106; Coleman, *The Irish sweep*, pp. 1–22.
99. Meath Hospital minute book, 31 August 1914 (NAI, 2007/128/5-3).
100. Durnin, 'Medicine in the city', pp. 83–106.
101. *Appendices to the report of the committee appointed to inquire into the extension of medical benefit under the National Insurance Act to Ireland* [Cd.7039], H.C. 1913, xxxvii, 64.
102. House of Industry hospitals minute book, 11 December 1914 (NAI, 2006/86).
103. *Irish Times*, 15 October 1918.
104. Book of Sir Patrick Dun's Hospital, 13 January 1915 (RCPI, PDH/1/2/1/9).
105. House of Industry hospitals minute book, 3 December 1915 (NAI, 2006/86).
106. House of Industry hospitals minute book, 17 December 1915 (NAI, 2006/86).
107. House of Industry hospitals minute book, 21 May 1915 (NAI, 2006/86).
108. Royal City of Dublin Hospital minute book, 8 October 1915 (NAI, 2006/98).
109. Figure based on calculations compiled from minute books of Dublin hospitals, including book of Sir Patrick Dun's Hospital (RCPI, PDH/1/2/1/9); House of Industry Hospital minute book (NAI, 2006/86); Royal City of Dublin Hospital minute book (NAI, 2006/98).
110. Peter Prime, *The history of the medical and hospital services of the Anglo-Boer War, 1899–1902* (Chester: Anglo-Boer War Philatelic Society, 1998), p. 57.
111. Royal City of Dublin Hospital minute book, 12 February 1915 (NAI, 2006/98).
112. Royal City of Dublin Hospital minute book, 11 June 1915 (NAI, 2006/98).
113. House of Industry hospitals minute book, 20 August 1915 (NAI, 2006/86).

114. Sir Patrick Dun's Hospital annual report, 1914 (RCPI, PDH/1/1/6-7).
115. Sir Patrick Dun's Hospital annual reports, 1914–1918 (RCPI, PDH/1/1/6-7).
116. Royal City of Dublin Hospital annual report, 1915 (NAI, 2006/98).
117. For more on wartime inflation, see Stephen Broadberry and Mark Harrison (eds.), *The economics of World War One* (Cambridge: Cambridge University Press, 2005).
118. Martin Kitchen, *Europe between the wars* (Harlow: Taylor & Francis, 2006), p. 55.
119. *Irish Times*, 24 July 1915.
120. Report of Deputy Director of Medical Services, Irish Command, 26 January 1920 (TNA, Irish situation, 1914–1922 collection, WO 35 179).
121. Royal City of Dublin Hospital minute book, 12 March 1915 (NAI, 2006/98).
122. *Belfast Newsletter*, 1 April 1916.
123. Figure based on calculations compiled from minute books of Dublin hospitals, including book of Sir Patrick Dun's Hospital (RCPI, PDH/1/2/1/9); House of Industry Hospital minute book (NAI, 2006/86); Royal City Dublin Hospital minute book (NAI, 2006/98).
124. *Fifty-seventh annual report of the Board of Superintendence of the Dublin Hospitals, with appendices* [Cd. 8030], H.C. 1916, XIV, 8.
125. *Fifty-seventh annual report of the Board of Superintendence of the Dublin Hospitals, with appendices* [Cd. 8030], H.C. 1916, XIV, 8.
126. Meath Hospital minute book, 11 January 1915 (NAI, 2007/128/5-3).
127. Gerard Fealy, *A history of apprenticeship nurse training in Ireland* (London: Routledge, 2005), p. 36.
128. Meath Hospital minute book, 4 January 1915 (NAI, 2007/128/5-3).
129. Meath Hospital minute book, 30 October 1916 (NAI, 2007/128/5-3).
130. Management committee book for Royal Victoria Hospital, 20 January 1915 (PRONI, MIC/514/1/1/21).
131. Meath Hospital minute book, 14 October 1918 (NAI, 2007/128/5-5).
132. House of Industry Hospitals minute book, 21 May 1915 (NAI, BR/2006/86).
133. Winter, 'Hospitals', p. 358.
134. Winter, 'Hospitals', p. 356.
135. Abel-Smith, *The hospitals*, p. 272.
136. Royal City of Dublin Hospital minute book, 11 December 1914 (NAI, 2006/98).
137. Royal City of Dublin Hospital minute book, 11 June 1915 (NAI, 2006/98).
138. Report of Deputy Director of Medical Services, Irish Command, 26 January 1920 (TNA, Irish situation, 1914–1922 collection, WO 35 179).
139. Sir Patrick Dun's Hospital annual report, 1916 (RCPI, PDH/1/1/7).

140. Account of soldiers treated at Royal Victoria Hospital, November 1914 (PRONI, HOS/2/1/4/1).
141. *Irish Times*, 25 March 1916.
142. Dublin Clinical Hospitals Committee correspondence, 11 December 1914 (RCPI, DCHC/2/14); Russell was appointed to the post during the war.
143. Letter from Secretary of Mater Misericordiae Hospital Medical Board, Dublin Clinical Hospitals Committee minute book, 5 December 1914 (RCPI, DCHC/2/15).
144. Sir Charles Ball and Thomas Myles to Dublin Clinical Hospitals Committee, 11 December 1914 (RCPI, DCHC/2/15).
145. Sir Charles Ball and Thomas Myles to Dublin Clinical Hospitals Committee, 11 December 1914 (RCPI, DCHC/2/15).
146. Dublin Clinical Hospitals Committee to Charles Ball and Thomas Myles, 12 December 1914 (RCPI, DCHC/2/15).
147. Dublin Clinical Hospitals Committee to Charles Ball and Thomas Myles, 12 December 1914 (RCPI, DCHC/2/15).
148. *Irish Times*, 14 January 1915.
149. *Medical Press*, 23 December 1914.
150. *Irish Times*, 17 Febraury 1915.
151. House of Industry Hospital minute book, 8 January 1915 (NAI, 2006/86).
152. Meath Hospital minute book, 30 October 1916 (NAI, 2007/128/5-3).
153. Meath Hospital minute book, 13 November 1916 (NAI, 2007/128/5-3).
154. Harrison, *The medical war*, p. 59.
155. Abel-Smith, *The hospitals*, p. 267.
156. Shephard, *A war of nerves*, p. 21.
157. Shephard, *A war of nerves*, p. 73.
158. Shephard, *A war of nerves*, p. 73.
159. Peter Barham, *Forgotten lunatics of the Great War* (New Haven: Yale University Press, 2007), p. 45.
160. Helen Andrews, 'Dawson, William Richard' in McGuire and Quinn (eds.), *Dictionary of Irish biography*, iii, 101.
161. W.R. Dawson, 'The work of the Belfast War Hospital' in *British Journal of Psychiatry*, 71 (1925), p. 219.
162. For more on the overcrowding of Irish asylums, see Catherine Cox, *Negotiating insanity in the southeast of Ireland, 1820–1900* (Manchester: Manchester University Press, 2012); Finnane, *Insanity and the insane in post-famine Ireland*, pp. 175–208.
163. Dawson, 'The work of the Belfast Hospital', p. 219.
164. Reynolds, *Grangegorman: Psychiatric care*, p. 192.

165. Reynolds, *Grangegorman: Psychiatric care*, p. 217; Peter Reid, 'The institutional management of soldiers with shell shock in Ireland, 1916–19' (MA thesis, University College, Dublin, 2014), p. 10.

166. *Richmond District Lunatic Asylum annual report of the medical superintendent*, 1917, p. 16 (NAI, uncatalogued).

167. Dawson, 'The work of the Belfast War Hospital', p. 219.

168. Lieutenant Colonel Hearn, RAMC, to R.M.S. Richmond Lunatic Asylum, Richmond War Hospital Admission and Discharge Book, 1 August 1916 (NAI, uncatalogued).

169. Shephard, *A war of nerves*, p. 73.

170. Barham, *Forgotten lunatics*, p. 45.

171. For more on lunatics in the workhouse, see Cox, *Negotiating insanity*, pp. 169–195; David Durnin, '"Intertwining institutions": The relationship between the South Dublin Union workhouse and the Richmond Lunatic Asylum, 1880–1911' (MA thesis, University College, Dublin, 2010).

172. *Irish Times*, 10 November 1917.

173. Dawson, 'The work of the Belfast War Hospital', p. 220.

174. Anon., 'Obituary: Lieut.-Colonel John Patrick Joseph Murphy, RAMC' in *British Medical Journal*, 3716, no. 1 (1932), p. 596.

175. Report of Deputy Director of Medical Services, Irish Command, 26 January 1920 (TNA, Irish situation, 1914–1922 collection, WO 35 179).

176. Roger Cooter, *Surgery and society in peace and war: Orthopaedics and the organisation of modern medicine, 1880–1948* (Basingstoke: Macmillan, 1993), p. 105.

177. Cooter, *Surgery and society*, p. 106.

178. Van Bergen, *Before my helpless sight*, p. 345.

179. *Irish Times*, 9 December 1916.

180. *Irish Times*, 9 December 1916.

181. *Irish Times*, 9 December 1916.

182. *Irish Times*, 12 December 1916.

183. *Irish Times*, 9 December 1916.

184. *Irish Times*, 7 July 1917.

185. *Irish Times*, 7 July 1917.

186. *Irish Independent*, 3 Febraury 1917.

187. *Belfast Newsletter*, 6 April 1917.

188. Report of Assistant Director of Medical Services, C&D Brigades, 9 December 1919 (TNA, Irish situation, 1914–1922 collection, WO 35 179).

189. Report of Assistant Director of Medical Services, C&D Brigades, 9 December 1919 (TNA, Irish situation, 1914–1922 collection, WO 35 179).

190. Report of Deputy Director of Medical Services, Irish Command, 26 January 1920 (TNA, Irish situation, 1914–1922 collection, WO 35 179).

191. Van Bergen, *Before my helpless sight*, p. 141.

192. Greta Jones, '*Captain of all these men of death*': *The history of tuberculosis in nineteenth and twentieth century Ireland* (Amsterdam: Rodopi, 2001), p. 128.
193. Report of Assistant Director of Medical Services, C&D Brigades, 9 December 1919 (TNA, Irish situation, 1914–1922 collection, WO 35 179).
194. *Kildare Observer*, 4 December 1915.
195. *Kildare Observer*, 4 December 1915.
196. Report of Assistant Director of Medical Services, C&D Brigades, 9 December 1919 (TNA, Irish situation, 1914–1922 collection, WO 35 179).
197. Jones, 'Captain of all these men of death', p. 130.
198. Harrison, *The medical war*, p. 228.
199. Harrison, *The medical war*, p. 233.
200. Report of Assistant Director of Medical Services, C&D Brigades, 9 December 1919 (TNA, Irish situation, 1914–1922 collection, WO 35 179); The exact number of sufferers is not provided by the report.
201. For more on VD and behaviour in Ireland, see Maria Luddy, 'Sex and the single girl in 1920s and 1930s Ireland' in *The Irish Review*, no. 35 (2007), pp. 79–91; Leanne McCormick, 'The dangers and temptations of the street: Managing female behaviour in Belfast during First World War' in *Women's History Review*, 27, no. 3, pp. 414–431.
202. Whitehead, *Doctors in the Great War*, p. 234.
203. *Royal Commission on Venereal Diseases: Final report of the commissioners*, [Cd. 8189], H.C. 1916, xci; Anon., 'The report of the Royal Commission on Venereal Diseases' in *British Medical Journal*, 2880, no. 1 (1916), p. 380.
204. Susannah Riordan, 'Venereal disease in the Irish Free State: The politics of public health' in *Irish Historical Studies*, 35, no. 139 (2007), p. 347.
205. Report of Assistant Director of Medical Services, 6th Division, 16 December 1919 (TNA, Irish situation, 1914–1922 collection, WO 35 179); *Freeman's Journal*, 23 November 1921. Dr. Steeven's Hospital was a notable exception as it admitted VD sufferers.
206. Report of Assistant Director of Medical Services, 6th Division, 16 December 1919 (TNA, Irish situation, 1914–1922 collection, WO 35 179).
207. *Freeman's Journal*, 16 March 1918.
208. *Irish Examiner*, 22 March 1918.
209. Report of Assistant Director of Medical Services, 6th Division, 16 December 1919 (TNA, Irish situation, 1914–1922 collection, WO 35 179); *Freeman's Journal*, 23 November 1921.
210. Harrison, *The medical war*, p. 65.
211. MacPherson, *History of the Great War*, p. 372. Between March and May 1917, there was a lull in the arrival of wounded in Ireland as no hospital

ships docked in Dublin. Lord Derby emphasised that the lack of hospital ship transports was due to a German campaign of submarine warfare. However, following this hiatus there was a rapid increase in the number of wounded returned to Ireland. See *Irish Times*, 28 April 1917.

212. See Appendix: Table C.
213. House of Industry Hospital minute book, 21 September 1917 (NAI, 2006/86).
214. House of Industry Hospital minute book, 7 December 1917 (NAI, 2006/86).
215. House of Industry Hospital minute book, 21 September 1917 (NAI, 2006/86).
216. House of Industry Hospital minute book, 4 May 1917 (NAI, 2006/86).
217. House of Industry Hospital minute book, 31 March 1917 (NAI, 2006/86).
218. Sir Patrick Dun's Hospital annual report, 1917 (RCPI, PDH/1/1/7).
219. Sir Patrick Dun's Hospital annual report, 1917 (RCPI, PDH/1/1/7).
220. Sir Patrick Dun's Hospital annual report, 1917 (RCPI, PDH/1/1/8).
221. Royal City of Dublin Hospital annual report, 1917 (NAI, 2006/98).
222. Fitzpatrick, 'Home front and everyday life', p. 35.
223. *Nationality*, 2 June 1917 cited in Ben Novick, *Conceiving revolution: Irish nationalist propaganda in the First World War* (Dublin: Four Courts Press, 2001), p. 66; *Nationality* was published 1915–1916 and 1917–1919 at the *Nationality* Office, D'Olier Street, Dublin. Edited by Arthur Griffith up to the time of his arrest in May 1918. Circulation of 8000. For more, see Carty, *Bibliography of Irish History, 1912–21*, p. 59. Griffith founded the *Sinn Féin* political party and was president of Dáil Éireann from January to August, 1922. For more, see Michael Laffan, 'Griffith, Arthur Joseph' in McGuire and Quinn (eds.), *Dictionary of Irish biography*, iv, 277.
224. Order of St. John of Jerusalem, *The Red Cross in Ireland*, p. 34.
225. The Royal Victoria Hospital had a history of receiving donations from unionists at the expense of donations to the Mater Hospital, Belfast (a Catholic institution). See Peter Martin, 'Why have a Catholic hospital at all? The Mater Infirmorum Hospital Belfast and the state, 1883–1972' in Donnacha Seán Lucey and Virginia Crossman (eds.), *Healthcare in Ireland and Britain from 1850* (London: Institute of Historical Research, 2014), p. 102.
226. *Belfast Newsletter*, 1 April 1916.
227. *Belfast Newsletter*, 1 April 1916.
228. *Belfast Newsletter*, 19 February 1918.
229. Donnacha Seán Lucey and George Campbell Gosling, 'Paying for health: Comparative perspectives on patient payment and contributions for

hospital provision in Ireland' in Lucey and Crossman (eds.), *Healthcare in Ireland and Britain from 1850*, p. 87.

230. *Belfast Newsletter*, 9 April 1918.
231. *Belfast Newsletter*, 9 April 1918.
232. Abel-Smith, *The hospitals*, p. 278.
233. Sir Patrick Dun's Hospital annual report, 1914 (RCPI, PDH/1/1/4).
234. Royal City of Dublin Hospital minute book, 11 May 1917 (NAI, 2006/98).
235. *Fifty-ninth annual report of the Board of Superintendence of the Dublin Hospitals, with appendices* [Cd. 8754], H.C. 1918, x.549, 4.
236. *Fifty-ninth annual report of the Board of Superintendence of the Dublin Hospitals, with appendices* [Cd. 8754], H.C. 1918, x.549, 5.
237. Fealy, *A history of apprenticeship nurse training*, p. 36.
238. *Belfast Newsletter*, 1 April 1916.
239. Several of these also served in the RAMC. For more, see *Medical Directory*, 1921.
240. House of Industry Hospital minute book, 5 April 1917 (NAI, 2006/86).
241. House of Industry Hospital minute book, 5 April 1917 (NAI, 2006/86).
242. Medical Staff Minute Book for the Royal Victoria Hospital, Belfast, 23 March 1915 (PRONI, MIC514/1/2/3).
243. Royal City of Dublin Hospital minute book, 12 April 1918 (NAI, 2006/98).
244. South Dublin Union Board of Guardians minute book, 12 June 1918 (NAI, MFGS 49/91).
245. South Dublin Union Board of Guardians minute book, 12 June 1918 (NAI, MFGS 49/91).
246. *Kildare Observer*, 13 February 1915.
247. *Irish Times*, 9 June 1916.
248. Anon., 'Dublin hospital Sunday' in *British Medical Journal*, 2939, no. 1 (1917), p. 563; The fund, founded in 1874, was controlled by a steering committee, elected each year, who organised various fundraising events throughout the year for the benefit of Dublin's voluntary hospitals. See Durnin, 'Medicine in the city', p. 90.
249. House of Industry Hospital minute book, 2 November 1917 (NAI, 2006/86).
250. North Dublin Union Board of Guardians minute book, 5 May 1915 (NAI, MFGS 49/128).

251. *Annual report of the Local Government Board for Ireland, for the year ended 31st March, 1915, being the forty-third report under the Local Government Board (Ireland) Act, 1872* [Cd. 8016] H.C. 1916, xxv.341, 30.

252. *Annual report of the Local Government Board for Ireland, for the year ended 31st March, 1915, being the forty-third report under the Local Government Board (Ireland) Act, 1872* [Cd. 8016] H.C. 1916, xxv.341, 30.

253. *Annual report of the Local Government Board for Ireland, for the year ended 31st March, 1915, being the forty-third report under the Local Government Board (Ireland) Act, 1872* [Cd. 8016] H.C. 1916, xxv.341, 30.

254. South Dublin Union Board of Guardians minute book, 12 March 1918 (NAI, MFGS 49/91).

CHAPTER 5

# British Army Medical Personnel in Post-war Ireland, 1918–1925

'To be in France during the war seems to me child's play compared with the conditions in Ireland, where you never know who is your friend'.[1]

On 11 November 1918, the Allies and Germany signed the Armistice of Compiegne signalling the end of hostilities in Western Europe. The War Office soon turned their attention to the process of demobilisation, which would return millions of enlisted soldiers in the British Army back to Britain and Ireland. By 1918, Britain had the largest functioning army, navy and air-force in the world, and the associated cost of maintaining the force in peacetime was too high to support.[2] Therefore, demobilisation needed to be achieved as quickly as possible but in a way that ensured a smooth transition for both military and civilian populations.[3] In 1917 Lord Derby, Secretary of State for War, proposed a demobilisation scheme.[4] Under the terms of this plan, men who held positions in key branches of industry were to be released from service first. This proposal, however, caused considerable unrest among long-serving soldiers who believed that those with the longest service records deserved to be demobilised before others. A new demobilisation scheme along these lines was proposed and adopted following Winston Churchill's appointment as Secretary of State for War in January 1919. By November 1919, the British Army had been reduced from 3.8 million men to approximately 900,000, and by 1922, just over 230,000 soldiers remained in the forces.[5]

© The Author(s) 2019                                               151
D. Durnin, *The Irish Medical Profession and the First World War*,
Medicine and Biomedical Sciences in Modern History,
https://doi.org/10.1007/978-3-030-17959-5_5

A corollary of military demobilisation was medical demobilisation, a process that this chapter will examine, together with an analysis of the difficulties that doctors encountered following their return to Ireland. Public support for the war had waned in Ireland, especially outside of Ulster, while Irish doctors were serving in the army. Fitzpatrick and Leonard have detailed the problems that Irish soldiers encountered when they returned from the war and found that many struggled to adapt to civilian life due to the domestic conflict—Irish War of Independence (January 1919–July 1921) and Irish Civil War (June 1922–May, 1923)—and hostility towards them from Sinn Féin and the IRA.[6] This chapter will question whether the experiences of returning medical personnel were similar to those of demobbed combatants and it will assess the role of doctors who participated in the First World War in Ireland's domestic conflicts.

Those who returned to Ireland after the war witnessed considerable political change in Ireland that was to influence employment structures for public medical appointments. Sinn Féin's victory in the 1918 general election led to the establishment of Dáil Éireann. Mary E. Daly has argued that the rise of militant nationalism which led to the founding of Dáil Éireann was slow to affect local government.[7] Dáil Éireann did not make any immediate effort to win the support of Irish local authorities—those responsible for public medical appointments—and were initially unsure as to whether guardians should continue to cooperate with the LGBI.[8] Nevertheless, Sinn Féin's growing influence on local government was evident by 1920. In January 1920 they gained control of 72 out of the 127 urban councils and county boroughs. The elections for the county councils, poor law boards and rural district councils were held in June and again, Sinn Féin candidates prospered.[9] As part of the wider political change, the Local Government (Temporary Provisions) Act 1923 and the 1925 Local Government Act resulted in the disbandment of boards of guardians and rural district councils in the Irish Free State. These were replaced by boards of health and public subsistence that were subsidiary to the county councils.[10] Doctors who participated in the First World War sought employment under this changing regime and as Daly notes, the merits of appointment were frequently assessed on the basis of religion or politics.[11]

Following the introduction of the Government of Ireland Act in 1920, there were also changes to public employment structures for doctors in Northern Ireland. The Act proposed separate home rule institutions within the six county Northern Ireland and a twenty-six county Southern Ireland. In Southern Ireland, candidates for election opted to assemble as Dáil Éireann rather than in the House of Commons but parliament commenced in Northern Ireland following elections in 1921. Under the terms of the Government of Ireland Act, the powers of the LGBI in Northern Ireland transferred to the Ministry of Home Affairs for Northern Ireland and this included the supervision of the several different forms of local administration such as the boards of guardians—those who controlled public medical appointments.[12] Alvin Jackson has argued that local authorities in Northern Ireland 'tended towards parsimony' in health and social welfare and that in the 1920s, the unionist administration 'did not have the political courage to challenge the vested interests of long-established local authorities'.[13] This chapter will investigate whether the political change in Ireland, north and south, influenced returning doctors' prospects of employment in public posts.

## MEDICAL DEMOBILISATION

From 1918, the Ministry of National Service, who oversaw the professional committees' medical recruitment drives during the latter stages of war, managed the demobilisation of medical personnel. The ministry established an interdepartmental committee, chaired by Sir James Galloway, Chief Commissioner of Medical Services in the Ministry of National Service, who had been a key member of the CMWC. Following the signing of the Armistice, the War Office altered the CMWC's purpose and instead, the group acted as advisors to the ministry on the demobilisation process. The CMWC created and proposed a scheme of demobilisation for army doctors and the ministry's interdepartmental committee adopted this. Under the terms of this arrangement, the first doctors to be demobilised were those with private practices, government or hospital posts in areas where medical services had been severely depleted. The CMWC and the ministry's committee then assessed the other medical personnel and demobilised them according to the length of their service, age, and family responsibilities. A special clause was also inserted in the demobilisation plan that allowed doctors with general practices to apply for quick release.[14]

As part of the demobilisation process, the committees considered the military's need for medical personnel as well as the requirements of the civilian population. Despite the signing of the armistice, the

British Army still maintained a presence in various locations abroad and therefore found it necessary to sustain a contingent of MOs and nurses in the army. Following the armistice, for instance, Michael Mahoney, a County Cork native who served in the RAMC during the conflict, was reposted to Northern Russia.[15] Catherine Black continued to nurse in France for months after the end of the war.[16] The ministry considered calling up recently qualified medical students to relieve doctors who had been on long-term active service. However, members of the medical profession, especially those involved in hospital work, objected to the proposal as it would deplete already impoverished levels of staffing at hospitals. In a letter to the *British Medical Journal* published in December 1918, Dr. Frank C. Eve, House-Physician in the Royal Infirmary, Hull, argued that 'everyone will sympathize with the object of this measure, but at the same time it will have to be carried out with great discretion if the work of the hospitals is not to be crippled for lack of house-physicians and house-surgeons. Already the supply of these is dangerously low'.[17]

The committees insisted that the men returning from war could fill the hospital positions. As shown, many newly qualified medical students had enlisted straight into the army without gaining experience on the wards and would have benefited from hospital work on their return. Dr. Herbert Butcher, a regular contributor to the letter pages of the *British Medical Journal*, argued that following demobilisation these men were anxious to hold resident appointments and many of them, on account of the nature of their military duties, had seen little of medicine or surgery for four years. Butcher emphasised that 'these officers should have a prior claim for resident hospital appointments to men who, although they have been doing most excellent work, have had it must be remembered, far better opportunities, in many cases of gaining professional experience'.[18]

The debates were moot. In April 1919, the War Office announced a wide-scale demobilisation of MOs from the RAMC to 'meet the pressing needs of the civilian population'.[19] As a result, from 1 April the Ministry of National Service no longer selected and nominated MOs for release. Instead, the War Office assumed control of the process. The War Office thus no longer required the CMWC and its subsidiary committees and the CMWC ceased operating in July.[20] The IMWC, however, continued to work throughout the summer of 1919; in May, the *British Medical Journal* reported that the IMWC was still 'working hard and made all the necessary inquiries in connection with the demobilisation of Irish doctors serving with the British military'.[21] The committee, which was to eventually disband later in the year, continued to function for a slightly longer period than the CMWC due to its role in securing doctors for the new Committee of Local Practitioners that had been formed in Ireland by the Ministry of National Service to work on the Review of Pensions Medical Boards.[22]

The demobilisation process for Irish medical personnel was similar to that of their British counterparts. Returning Irish doctors departed their assigned posts abroad and travelled to various reception ports, including Southampton, and then officially demobilised at a dispersal centre. Dr. James Abraham was demobilised and travelled from Alexandria to England. He recounted his experience of official demobilisation, which involved a visit to a dispersal centre where he was 'issued with what was called a protection certificate which said I was disembodied with effect from April. It sounded bad, but I felt no ill effects, and decided I could now go home to my family in Ulster'.[23]

Several different factors encouraged the War Office to abolish the medical committees and swiftly return doctors to Ireland and Britain. Adam Seipp has argued that the demobilisation process, as a whole, was dizzyingly complex and that in some cases it appeared to lack any planning at all.[24] The swift demobilisation of doctors was somewhat reckless as it reintroduced a large number of doctors into the civilian medical profession with little consideration for civilian medical infrastructure. Yet, the cost of maintaining a large RAMC force in peacetime motivated the War Office to release doctors. While the British Army required doctors in various regions in the years after the war, ultimately, the large force that had been accumulated during the First World War was unnecessary and considerably costly.

The War Office's release of MOs also coincided with the increasing demand for doctors in both Britain and Ireland due to the outbreak of influenza. Anne Rasmussen has argued that the influenza epidemic touched every region of the world in the brief and concentrated period of 1918–1919.[25] As Caitriona Foley has demonstrated, influenza struck Ireland in three waves—spring 1918 to July 1918; September to November 1918; and early spring 1919.[26] The timing of the outbreak in Ireland was linked to the return of demobilised soldiers, as the disease spread in areas with high recruitment rates—the province of Ulster and the counties of Dublin, Wicklow, Carlow and Kildare.[27]

On 7 December 1918, the *Irish Independent* claimed that the 'prevalence of the influenza epidemic is considered a special reason why as many army doctors and nurses as possible should be demobilised without delay'.[28] According to separate studies by Foley, Ida Milne and Patricia Marsh, 'civilising institutions' were among the worst hit by influenza and the inhabitants of workhouses, mental hospitals and national schools suffered.[29] The workhouse system was particularly badly hit, with institutions in Cork, Donegal, Dublin, Galway and Wicklow reporting high rates of infection and of mortality.[30] With large numbers of workhouse medical staff serving in the British Army, it was unsurprising that guardians were calling to have their MOs returned from war. Poor law guardians in several of these areas urgently requested additional MOs to treat the large number of influenza sufferers.[31] In October 1918, Alderman O'Toole, a member of the Dublin Corporation, bemoaned at a meeting of the Dublin Board of Guardians, that they had 'great difficulty in getting doctors. In fact they had to ask the clerk to hunt round the city to get three medical men to take the place of others and give assistance'.[32]

In several poor law unions, the guardians and local RAMC Command reached an agreement whereby the RAMC would provide medical support to the local workhouse infirmaries until other medical staff was secured. In December 1918, prior to the general medical demobilisation, the Clones Board of Guardians in County Monaghan approached the RAMC for assistance in dealing with the influenza outbreak in their union and consequently the RAMC sent eight of their members from their base in Belfast to the Clones workhouse infirmary. Influenza patients had overcrowded the infirmary. According to the guardians, RAMC medical personnel 'remained on duty night and day for the space of two or three weeks'.[33] This provided some short-term support to overworked poor-law medical staff and demonstrated cooperation between RAMC and civilian medical staff but it was not a long-term solution to the shortage of medical staff in Irish poor law unions.

In the period between the Armistice and wide-scale demobilisation of doctors, boards of guardians wrote to the War Office requesting the swift release of their dispensary and workhouse MOs to bolster their medical staffs. At a meeting of the Ballymahon Board of Guardians in County Longford, for instance, P. McCormack, a member of the board, declared that 'we want a doctor here in Ballymahon very badly'.[34] The guardians resolved to write to the War Office requesting the return of Dr. Charles Kenny, a MO from the area who had enlisted in the RAMC. Kenny soon demobilised and returned to Ballymahon Workhouse.[35] The War Office encouraged guardians to communicate with them as part of the demobilisation process but it was evident in several cases that Irish boards of guardians were unaware that their requests could expediate the release of their doctors. Dr. Charles Bryan, who had been a MO in Kiltegan dispensary district in County Wicklow before temporarily enlisting in the RAMC, had to inform the local board of guardians in Baltinglass that the question of his release from the RAMC 'should emanate from the board of guardians itself'.[36] The LGBI offered some support to the guardians during this process. In December 1918 the LGBI informed the Castlederg Board of Guardians in County Tyrone that it had recommended the War Office to accede to the guardians' request to discharge Major Leary from the RAMC so that he could return to his role as MO in the Castlederg dispensary district.[37]

Despite this assistance, guardians were largely critical of the LGBI because it maintained its right to veto appointments of medical practitioners of war age to dispensary posts during the initial demobilisation phase.[38] Ida Milne has posited that the official response in Ireland to the influenza epidemic, like elsewhere in Britain and internationally, was slow.[39] The LGBI's refusal to ease its wartime employment restrictions on medical posts in the midst of the influenza epidemic supports this thesis. From the signing of the Armistice until March 1919, the LGBI continually refused to sanction the appointments of young doctors despite the crippling shortage of medical staff during the influenza outbreak. For example, in January 1919 the LGBI refused to sanction the permanent appointment of Dr. William Lane as MO at the Castletown dispensary in County Kildare. The LGBI explained that 'until young medical men now temporarily serving with his majesty's forces were demobilised and in a position to offer themselves as candidates for appointment in the poor law medical service, the Board were not willing to sanction the filling up permanently of vacancies in that service'.[40] The Castletown Board of Guardians resolved to 'fight the matter out with the LGBI'.[41] Other boards simply ignored the LGBI's ruling. When appointing a MO to the Coolock and Drumcondra dispensary, the North Dublin Board of Guardians decided to 'not take any dictation from the LGBI and ignore their letter'.[42] It was not until the end of March 1919, following the War Office's wide-scale demobilisation of MOs from the British Army medical services, that the LGBI informed guardians that it had 'formally withdrawn the prohibition ...

of November 1915' and guardians could once again appoint permanent MOs to available posts.[43]

## THE RETURN OF IRELAND'S BRITISH ARMY DOCTORS, 1918–1925

Following the War Office's large demobilisation of MOs from the British Army medical services and the LGBI's removal of their employment veto, demobbed medical personnel sought work.[44] Firstly, not all returned to Ireland. In a return to pre-war trends, many secured employment in Britain and further afield. Following a brief holiday in Ireland, Catherine Black returned to nurse in a London hospital.[45] There are countless other examples of Irish wartime nurses who relocated to Britain after the war. A similar trend was evident among Ireland's wartime doctors. Benson, assistant surgeon at Sir Patrick Dun's Hospital, argued that 'the industrial districts of England will be able to offer financial attractions to doctors quite beyond those obtainable in very many of the dispensary districts in Ireland'.[46] Numerous demobbed Irish doctors established private practices or secured hospital posts in Britain. Francis Crosbie, a TCD graduate who had worked in the National Hospital for Consumption for Ireland prior to enlisting in the RAMC, established a general practice in the London borough of Ealing.[47] John Green, who had joined the RAMC prior to the outbreak of war, secured hospital appointments in London and Wolverhampton, set up a private practice in Monmouth, and then went to practise in Worthing.[48] There are copious other examples.[49]

While a medical career in Britain was an attractive prospect for the demobbed Irish doctor, it was often difficult for doctors to establish or re-establish practices there due to the competitive nature of the British medical profession. Following his demobilisation from Alexandria in Egypt, James Abraham went to England in March 1919. Abraham had been a surgeon in a west London hospital before the war and he had rented consulting rooms in the city for a private practice. In 1916 he had let the rooms go 'after seeing no prospect of the war ever ending'.[50] On Abraham's return to London, he attempted to secure new consulting rooms, but it was more difficult than he expected, as there were few spaces available. According to Abraham, the 'men who had been in France, and acquired surgical status there, had got back before me.

Men who had dodged the war, and had managed to worm their way into positions and practices when we were on active service, had no intention of being pushed out. This was depressing'.[51] He was eventually able to return to surgery in the West London Hospital, where he had worked prior to enlisting in the RAMC.[52] Abraham's hospital work thus provided him with a re-entry into the British medical profession but not all doctors who returned from war had hospital appointments to return to and others were forced to relocate to secure a profitable practice or post.

Other doctors who had participated in the war utilised their wartime experience and pursued careers in the RAMC, IMS and Royal Navy. Those who returned from temporary wartime commissions in the services and sought to continue were more likely to continue on temporary commissions that lasted for one year or until the War Office no longer required their services, with a rate of pay of £550 per annum in the RAMC.[53] Doctors who had held permanent posts in the British Army medical services prior to the war, including Stafford Adye-Curran and J. P. Lynch, continued their service in the post-war years and advanced their careers. Richard Hingston continued in the IMS and commanded military hospitals in various European countries. In 1924, he was also MO for the British Mount Everest Expedition.[54] Several other Irish doctors rose to the very top of the British military medical services. Joseph Chambers, a County Cavan native, who graduated from TCD, entered the navy in 1889 and served throughout the First World War. In 1923, he succeeded Sir Robert Hill as Director General of the British Army medical department. Likewise, Thomas Gallwey, who was born in County Waterford and educated at QUB, continued in the RAMC at the end of hostilities and in 1921 was appointed Colonel-Commandant. He had entered the Army medical department as surgeon in 1874, retired from the RAMC in 1911 but returned to serve in the war.

For those that returned to Ireland, their association with the RAMC assisted in their search for employment in posts related to British Army work. Ex-RAMC doctors who returned to Ireland were well placed to take advantage of the limited opportunities associated with the treatment of ex-soldiers. Jessica Meyer has suggested that by 1929, approximately 1,600,000 men were in receipt of pensions from the British government for disabilities incurred during the war.[55] The Ministry of Pensions (MOP), established in 1916, administered the assessment and payment of pensions to invalided combatants. In Britain, panel doctors treated demobilised impaired men but in Ireland, the panel-doctor system was not in operation. Instead, the MOP arranged directly with local medical practitioners to assess soldiers.[56] In 1918, the MOP authorised the Irish Insurance Commissioners to organise a scheme for the treatment of invalided soldiers, which included the provision of a general practitioner and medicine. The wounded had the right to choose their own practitioner and often selected local doctors who had served in the army.[57]

Medical referees, who certified whether patients required treatment, first attended to demobilised men.[58] Initially these medical referees were local doctors who were tasked with identifying the extent of the soldiers' injuries and the veracity of their claims. It was their duty to spot malingerers.[59] Bourke has suggested that the MOP was suspicious of Irish soldiers and required medical referees to be both precise in their diagnosis and awareness of wartime injuries.[60] In 1919, the House of Commons appointed a Select Committee on Pensions, chaired by Sir Montague Barlow, to report on the method of administering the pensions' acts. During their discussions on Ireland, the committee deliberated on the method of appointment of medical referees. W. G. Fallon, Secretary of the Local War Pensions Committee Dublin, expressed concern that medical referees in Dublin were appointed without any consultation with members of his committee and instead, were selected by the MOP and the Irish branch of the BMA. Sir John Butcher and Major Entwistle, members of a House of Commons' committee, encouraged the appointment of ex-army doctors as medical referees, stating that 'as you are aware, there are a great many of those civilians who joined the army who came back after four years and found their practice destroyed; these are the sort of men, if competent, one would like to give priority to'.[61] Subsequently, the MOP employed several ex-RAMC doctors to act as medical referees. For example, Henry Harbison, an NUI graduate from County Derry, who had served with the RAMC with distinction in France and was awarded the Croix de Guerre, secured a post as the MOP medical referee for Dublin. Harold Saunderson Sugars, the Irish rugby international and former RAMC doctor, was another ministry-appointed medical referee. During the war, he was attached to a battalion of the Yorkshire Light Infantry and was awarded the Military Cross. Following the Armistice, he was appointed as the MOP's Principal Officer in Ireland.[62]

RAMC veterans encouraged Irish medics who had returned from the war to emphasise their military experience when searching for work. Among those seeking employment, were returning army surgeons. The post-First World War period was not the first time that a large cohort of Irish surgeons returned from war looking for work in a highly competitive domestic medical marketplace. A contingent of army surgeons returned to Ireland following service in the Revolutionary and Napoleonic Wars. Ackroyd et al., have argued that those military surgeons were well placed to succeed in the medical profession following their demobilisation.[63] Similarly, Whitehead has contended that army surgeons benefited from improved surgical skills because of their time in the military during the First World War.[64] Speaking at the Royal Victoria Hospital's annual meeting in 1919, Andrew Fullerton, Belfast surgeon and colonel in the RAMC, stressed that many of the medical lessons learned at war would be 'of inestimable benefit in civil practice, especially in places like Belfast, in which unfortunately shock and haemorrhage from industrial accidents were all too common'.[65]

While Fullerton's argument was valid, it is important not to overstate the benefits of surgical skills gained during conflict. As Cooter has observed, medical developments during the First World War were, for the most part, not necessarily maintained or indeed useful in civilian medical practice.[66] For most Irish doctors returning from war, war surgery was quite different from surgery in a civilian hospital and the skills earned in wartime were of little benefit. Following his return to a hospital post, James Abraham was shocked to see that his first operation was on a woman suffering from breast cancer. He proclaimed 'good lord, I haven't operated on a woman for years, wonder if I'll remember'.[67]

Nonetheless, it was important for demobbed Irish medics to emphasise any relevant experience gained while applying for jobs due to the increased competition for posts in the Irish medical profession. Following the end of the war, the number of doctors seeking employment swiftly outstripped the availability of hospital and poor law posts in Ireland. Doctors who had their jobs kept open for them while they were at war returned to their careers. Others who had lost their job or practice during their wartime service, or had been newly qualified on enlistment, embarked upon a search for work in a medical profession that was even more overcrowded than it had been in the years that immediately preceded war. According to the *Medical Directory* published in 1920, the number of registered doctors in Ireland had increased from 2897 in 1914 to 3322 in 1918. As shown in Table 5.1, this was the largest percentage increase in the number of registered doctors across any of the regions recorded in the directory.

**Table 5.1**    Number of registered doctors, 1914–1918

| Year | London | Provinces | Wales | Scotland | Ireland | Abroad |
|---|---|---|---|---|---|---|
| 1914 | 6604 | 17,837 | 1402 | 4032 | 2897 | 5844 |
| 1915 | 6715 | 18,109 | 1415 | 4070 | 2981 | 5916 |
| 1916 | 6821 | 18,216 | 1433 | 4173 | 3060 | 5593 |
| 1917 | 6903 | 18,186 | 1445 | 4334 | 3193 | 5615 |
| 1918 | 6903 | 18,090 | 1447 | 4482 | 3322 | 5646 |
| % Increase 1914–1918 | 4.5 | 1.4 | 3.2 | 11.2 | 14.7 | –3.4 |

*Source* Numbers compiled from *Medical Directory*, 1920

There were several causes for the rise. Students had continued to graduate from Ireland's medical schools during the conflict, adding to the number of qualified doctors. Many had established private practices in the latter years of the war in regions previously served by general practitioners enlisted in the RAMC. This was a particular worry for demobbed army doctors. On 27 June 1919, an anonymous demobilised medic wrote a letter to the *British Medical Journal*:

> I, like the majority of medical officers while serving temporarily in the army or navy, heard on all sides about the great shortage and urgent need for doctors in civilian work. But on being demobilized, I find to my surprise that (I am only speaking for my own town) there is no shortage of doctors at all – on the contrary these is an increase, and yet there are large numbers of medical officers still being retained with the troops, both at home and abroad. Apart from this, there are also those who can never return, having given up their lives for their country, but whose absence should still further increase this shortage. I understand that I am by no means alone in this experience, and that doctors who have served are now finding out on their return that, with only the nucleus of their old practices left, they have to face the opposition of new-comers, who have already comfortably established themselves in the immediate neighbourhood.[68]

Among these students were those who, once qualified, were declared physically unfit for war service and thus secured temporary medical posts in various dispensaries for the duration of the war. Doctors who returned from war were often at a disadvantage compared to this contingent in the competition for public medical posts. Within weeks of the LGBI removing its veto on permanent medical appointments, multiple boards of guardians permanently appointed doctors who had held temporary MO posts during the war. In April 1919, the Dublin Guardians permanently appointed Drs P. E. Harrington and Andrew Ryan, who had held temporary MO positions during the war.[69] In the Stamullen Dispensary District in County Meath, Dr. J. A. Lynch, who had served as temporary MO for more than two years during the war, secured the post permanently following the removal of the veto.[70] Similarly, the Listowel Board of Guardians in County Kerry permanently appointed Dr. Conor Martin as the MO of the Ballylongford dispensary district; Martin had been temporarily appointed to the position in 1917.[71]

In addition, a significant number of women entered the profession during the war and offered considerable competition for returning army doctors searching for employment.[72] As Laura Kelly posits, women doctors became a crucial component of Ireland's medical infrastructure during the war years and they were keen to continue with their professional careers, further increasing the number of doctors in search of work.[73] In the post-war period, women doctors accepted lower financial terms than their male counterparts to establish themselves in public posts. In September 1922, at a meeting of the Dublin Board of Guardians, several candidates who had applied for the post of an MO in the Rathdown Union in County Dublin informed the board that they were withdrawing their applications due to the low salary on offer. It emerged that fellow medical professionals had informed the applicants that they would be regarded as 'letting down their professional brethren by not insisting on increased remuneration' for the post. However, two female applicants—Drs. Carmel Farrell and Annie Scully—refused to withdraw their applications. Scully was called before the guardians and she told them that she was 'in a very awkward position, inasmuch as she was informed that the other doctors had declared that they would not work with her'. She told the board that she considered the salary an 'adequate one, and much more than she was receiving, although she was a first-class honours student … she had worked as well as she possibly could, and personally did not care whether she got the position or not, but she had worked in a straightforward way for it'.[74] Scully was appointed to the post. That there was still competition for public medical jobs despite the low salary on offer was indicative of the struggle for work in the Irish medical profession.

The arguments over the salary offered for MO work was not unique to the Rathdown Union. Demobbed doctors returned to Ireland in the midst of rising disputes regarding salary for dispensary posts and their return escalated MOs' demands for a fairer salary. Remuneration for state positions was so low—the rate of pay had remained the same for many years but the cost of living had increased considerably due to war— that poor law MOs in several unions throughout the country, including Ballymena, Cavan, Coleraine, Dublin and Dundalk threatened to, or went on, strike.[75] In a dispute that was typical of others throughout Ireland, dispensary doctors in Enniskillen Union, County Fermanagh, resigned from their posts and declared that they would not resume duty until the guardians increased the doctors salaries by fifty per cent and introduced an annual increment.[76] Dr. Thomas Hennessy, Secretary of the Irish Medical Association, met with boards of guardians in almost every union regarding pay for dispensary doctors and MOs. At a meeting of the Nenagh Board of Guardians in County Tipperary, Hennessy argued that the salary scale for MOs—£170 to £220—was outdated and did not reflect their work. It also compared unfavourably with salary scales for other medical posts. He insisted that the scale was particularly unsuitable for doctors who had returned from war:

> army authorities were offering between £600 and £700 per year to doctors just qualified ... Irish doctors were paid by the Indian Medical Service £700 and £800 a year simply for treating Blacks ... If an Irish doctor selected to live in his own country he was sure they [the guardians] would make it worth his while and that he would not have to go elsewhere.[77]

In his request for a salary increase from the Abbeyleix Board of Guardians, Dr. Thomas Dunne also referred to the money available in the British Army medical services: 'The LG Board insisted – rightly I maintain – that all young doctors should join the army, therefore why not give us army pay now?'.[78] In a letter to the *British Medical Journal*, a disabled veteran doctor simply described the salaries offered to doctors, as 'so miserably small that it would not tempt a rat-catcher in his own profession'.[79]

By 1920, 146 of the 154 boards of guardians in Ireland had granted improved remuneration—either increased salaries or higher scales—to their MOs. Most of the new scales were fixed at a maximum of £250 per annum.[80] Yet for MOs in larger dispensary districts, these salary scales were still wholly inadequate. On 24 March 1920, Drs. Dillon, O'Reilly and Murnane informed the Dunshauglin Board of Guardians in County

Meath that they had rejected an offer from the LGBI to raise their salaries to £365 per year. The doctors noted that they would not accept anything less than £400 for working in their large dispensary districts. In a letter to the LGBI they stated that

> unless we are dealt with fairly we cannot continue to perform our work and must cease until such time as we are paid a reasonable living wage. To deny us that and expect us to continue at work is a mean effort to trade on the philanthropic humanity of the medical profession.[81]

Similarly, twelve MOs of the Rathdown Union, prior to the appointment of Dr. Scully, threatened to resign after the LGBI rejected their demands for an increased salary scale. The LGBI responded that the maximum salary of £300 a year, which had been recently raised, was payment for part of their time only and that this did not preclude them from 'engaging in extensive private practice ... the Board also would have thought that some of the medical officers of the Rathdown Union might have realised that in resorting to personal abuse (towards LGBI members) they (have not) strengthened their claims for further increases of salary'.[82] Members of the LGBI insisted that some of the Rathdown MOs had verbally abused them at a public function. The LGBI also explained that should the MOs resign.

> the Board will be prepared to make suggestions to the Guardians for the amalgamation of the posts as an alternative to filling up the twelve vacancies by which they believe it will be possible to carry on the medical services of the dispensaries, and the workhouse with very considerable economy to the ratepayers and with equal efficiency so far as the interests of the sick poor are concerned and upon terms as regards salaries which will secure the Guardians a wide choice of applicants.[83]

In response, Thomas Hennessy argued that in one of the Rathdown dispensary districts there were 2185 insured people and practically all of them, with their dependants, received medical treatment when ill as poor-law patients from the dispensary doctor. For treating this number of insured, 'a doctor in England was paid £1200 per annum', far above the maximum £300 allowed to the Rathdown MOs.[84] Despite these appeals, disputes regarding the MO salary in Rathdown continued without a satisfactory conclusion for most of the doctors until the LGBI's departure from Ireland.

## POLITICAL CHANGE IN IRELAND[85]

Demobilised Irish doctors faced several other difficulties in their search for employment including the tense and changing political landscape in Ireland. Soldiers who returned to Ireland after participating in the war complained of receiving abuse and threats in Ireland due to their association with the British Army. In his evidence to the Select Committee on Pensions, W. G. Fallon claimed that:

> A reaction took place in Dublin in this sense, that these men went off amidst the enthusiasm of the public in Dublin four or five years ago. There was tremendous enthusiasm and applause and God-speeds, but in the intervening period things happened in Ireland, and when these men came back disabled and broken down in some cases they found that their own relatives had changed their views on public affairs, and matters were exceedingly uncomfortable for the unfortunate man. I do not quite know whether I ought to mention this at all, but difficulties have not yet been overcome in Ireland and are only too evident.[86]

In the 1980s, Jane Leonard interviewed several Irish First World War veterans and some of those recalled hostile reactions towards them when they returned to Ireland. One interviewee, Jack Campbell, recalled an incident after his discharge from the King George V Hospital:

> When I came back, I couldn't get out of Dublin quick enough. I tell you this, I got discharged, as I told you, from the King George V Hospital on the 28[th] August. One evening I was in uniform. I was walking down Westmoreland Street … I noticed two ladies, well I won't call them ladies. Two women and two men were coming towards me and when they got alongside me, the two women stepped over in front of me and spit [sic] on me. That was their way of saying they didn't like British soldiers. They didn't ask me if I was Irish or Dutch or what. I thought to myself, I don't know. There was no work here and certainly there wasn't any work for the ex-British servicemen because they weren't liked … I got out of Dublin quick and went over to England. And I didn't come back to Dublin until I was retired and seventy years old … The couple of ladies spitting on me didn't leave any doubt in my mind where I wanted to go. Wanted to go back, you know, where I had respect.[87]

Likewise, Fitzpatrick has established that veterans, including those in the first batch of demobilised men, were intimidated by letters, assaulted and their homes and workplaces were subject to arson attacks.[88] Returning medics recounted tales of intimidation. In 1918, Abraham, a Coleraine native, returned to Ulster to visit his family following his service in the RAMC. He retained his uniform and he continued to wear it following his demobilisation. He noted that while travelling to Fermanagh to visit an uncle:

> everyone was friendly as far as Enniskillen; but when I got out at the station at Lisnaskea, [County Fermanagh] a man on the platform looked at my uniform, scowled and spat on the ground. This upset me. I knew nothing much of the Casement Rising, the trouble in 1916, and the bitterness that followed; but I was now practically on the border between the warring factions, and obviously feelings were still acute. It gave me a curiously unpleasant jolt. Things were clearly very different.[89]

In separate studies, Leonard and Eunan O'Halpin have examined the death rates of ex-servicemen in post-war Ireland. Leonard has estimated that between the beginning of the war and July 1921, the date of truce in the Irish War of Independence, approximately eighty-two ex-British Army soldiers were killed in Ireland.[90] O'Halpin has determined that approximately one-half of civilians killed as spies during the War of Independence and its aftermath were ex-servicemen.[91]

In his analysis of veterans' return to Ireland, Paul Taylor has argued that the IRA primarily targeted ex-soldiers for reasons other than their war service.[92] Medical veterans' experiences partly support this claim. While not victims of assassination, some ex-British army doctors were subject to intense intimidation because they attended to hunger strikers. Perhaps the most notable case of this occurred in County Cork where Dr. Alan Pearson attended hunger strikers in Cork prison. Pearson was an English doctor who had served in France during the war. Three days after he took the job in Cork, Pearson received a letter from the IRA notifying him that should any of the men in the jail die then he would be held accountable and killed. Two days later he received another letter ordering him to leave the jail at once and the country within twenty-four hours. He withdrew from attending the strikers but continued working in Cork prison for ten weeks before returning to England. He left Cork under armed escort before departing to England on the *HMS Heather*. Pearson stated that he would not 'for a hundred pounds day' go through the experience again.[93] As William Murphy has established, several MOs involved in forcible feeding of nationalist prisoners were intimidated.[94] The intimidation of Pearson was due to his role in Cork prison rather than his veteran status.

Nonetheless, it is not possible, at least in the case of doctors, to agree wholly with Taylor's assertion that British Army veterans were 'not marginalised in Irish society'.[95] There is some evidence that Irish doctors who participated in the war had to overcome some guardians' negative perceptions of wartime service to secure public medical appointments. In several districts, primarily in Northern Ireland, boards of guardians valued doctors' wartime service when appointing new dispensary doctors. When the Ballymoney Board of Guardians in County Antrim appointed Dr. John Warwick as MO for their dispensary district, they acknowledged his 'distinguished war service' during the appointment process.[96] Yet in the immediate post-war years, Sinn Féin controlled most of the boards of guardians and in several instances these boards discriminated against those who had served in the British Army. Doctors were aware of this. When looking for a position as MO at a Tipperary dispensary district, Dr. Richard Hennessy, who qualified from the NUI shortly before enlisting in the RAMC, requested that his neighbour Tom Kavanagh:

> use influence with Martin and John Meagher on my behalf. Dr. Powell of Roscrea is about to resign – and I'm going for his job. I don't think somehow the Meaghers are in my favour since I went out to France but I'd have gone just the same at that time if the Japs and Chinese were at it. Besides my work was an act of mercy. But you never know in what light some of the Guardians may look at it. In any case I want their [the Meaghers] support if I am to win so I shall rely on you to do all in your power for me.[97]

The Meaghers were members of the boards of guardians in Tipperary. John Meagher was chairman of the guardians in Roscrea Union. Martin Meagher was a nationalist and was close friends with Séamus Bourke who had been elected Sinn Féin T. D.—member of Dáil Éireann—for mid-Tipperary in 1918.[98] Hennessy did not secure the post. Instead, he continued to work in a private practice in Templemore before eventually becoming the MO of Borris-in-Ossory dispensary in nearby County Laois in 1923, shortly after the end of the Civil War.[99]

Of course, it is difficult to say whether Hennessy did not secure the post in Tipperary because of his service in the RAMC but there is evidence elsewhere of other guardians' open hostility towards doctors who served in the First World War. In November 1919, three doctors—Drs. Michael Sexton, Thomas Ryan and Joseph F. O'Regan—applied to the Cork Board of Guardians for the position of MO for the Carrigaline dispensary district in County Cork. The guardians appointed Dr. Ryan to the post, noting that 'his grandfather had been chairman [of the board of guardians] for a quarter of a century'.[100] Despite Ryan's strong family connection, some members of the board resisted his appointment due to his wartime service in the RAMC. In a thinly-veiled criticism of doctors who enlisted during the war, Mr J. Lane, a member of the board, urged support for Dr. Sexton because he had 'remained in their service and attended to their poor while other gentlemen went and earned the highest penny from the British Government'.[101] J Good, another member of the board, argued that 'he knew men who were in the army and they were good Irishmen, but so long as Prussian methods were applied to this country the Irishmen who worked for the British Government should be paid by the British Government'.[102] Mr T. Kiely, the guardian who had proposed Ryan's election, was compelled to defend the doctor's wartime service and argued that Ryan had applied for a dispensary post elsewhere prior to enlisting but had been defeated by a small number of votes and 'he would not have worn the khaki if he had been elected then but he had to go where he could earn a living'.[103] In this case, Dr. Ryan got the post due to his strong family ties with the Cork Board of Guardians but it is evident from the debates surrounding his appointment that doctors who had enlisted with the RAMC during wartime had to overcome some guardians' negative opinions towards those who had participated in the war to secure dispensary jobs.

Elsewhere in Ireland, doctors who returned to the dispensary posts that they had held before securing temporary leave to participate in war sometimes experienced fractious relationships with the local boards of guardians due to their wartime service. Issues arose before the doctors returned from war. In 1919, several boards issued ultimatums to doctors who continued to serve in the RAMC to either return to their dispensaries or resign their positions. In County Wicklow, the Baltinglass Board of Guardians requested Dr. Charles H. Bryan, who was serving with the 6th Field Ambulance, to relinquish his temporary commission in the RAMC or resign as MO to the Kiltegan district. Bryan responded that the guardians should be aware that 'the war did not terminate till the peace terms had been ratified'.[104] Bryan eventually returned to Kiltegan but experienced further problems with the guardians a year later due to his decision to treat the British military in Baltinglass—outside of his dispensary duties, Bryan was a temporary MO for the RAMC, treating British forces in the locality. In September 1920, the Board of Guardians demanded that Bryan stop attending the British forces. Bryan acquiesced to the guardians' request but noted that he regarded the action of the Board as an 'infringement of the right duty of every medical man at all times under all circumstances to attend all sick and wounded when requested to do so, at least in any civilised or Christian country. The resolution was also, in his opinion, an interference with the doctors' right to private practice'.[105] Bryans' strained relationship with the Baltinglass guardians was just one exemplar of a common scenario for demobbed British Army doctors in Ireland after the First World War; boards of guardians opposed to British rule were often hostile towards medical personnel who had served in the RAMC and threatened their careers as dispensary MOs if these doctors sought to continue their relationship with the British Army beyond the end of the First World War.

The employment problems of demobbed doctors who returned to the provinces outside of Ulster were compounded by the fact that the medical associations that often lobbied on their behalf were disrupted by political change and conflict in Ireland. In Ulster, a medico-political committee was formed under the Northern Parliament. The Ulster Committee included representation from Ulster medical committees and other medical organisations, as well as the branches of the British and Irish medical associations. This committee informed the Northern Government on medical matters and represented the medical profession in the six counties.[106] In contrast, the medical profession elsewhere in Ireland struggled to meet with any regularity to discuss the matters that concerned them. On 3 June 1919, a meeting of delegates, representative of the whole medical profession in Ireland, was held in Dublin to appoint a Joint Organisation Committee (Ireland), consisting of five members of the Irish Medical Association; five members of the British Medical Association and five members of the Irish Medical Committee (a body representing the whole medical profession in Ireland, including the medical schools). The Irish medical profession tasked the Joint Organisation Committee to consider the question of uniting the Irish medical profession into one representative organisation for all of Ireland. The greater part of the BMA's Irish medico-political work during the immediate post-world war years was done through the composite body of the Irish Medical Committee whose secretarial duties were discharged in an honorary capacity jointly by the Irish Medical Secretary of the British Medical Association and the Secretary of the Irish Medical Association.[107] However, the committee struggled to meet with any regularity until 1925 due to the domestic conflict, or what the committee termed 'the very disturbed condition of the country'.[108]

## EX-BRITISH ARMY DOCTORS AND CONFLICT IN IRELAND[109]

Demobbed Irish doctors participated in the Irish War of Independence and Civil War. The IRA often utilised doctors who had served in the RAMC because they had experience of treating gunshot wounds and could thus provide appropriate medical treatment to members of the IRA.[110] These doctors assisted for three reasons—it was their professional duty to tend to the sick and wounded; some were subject to intimidation, and others supported the aims of the IRA. William O'Hora, member of the IRA North Mayo Brigade called on a former British Army doctor to treat a wounded member of his company. O'Hora warned the doctor of 'the consequences of revealing details of what he had learned'. Faced with this threat, the doctor agreed to help and assured O'Hora 'that professional etiquette would not permit him to divulge anything like that'.[111]

In contrast, Thomas Myles, who had been the RAMC's consultant surgeon in Ireland, was not subjected to threats but willingly assisted the IRA because he supported their aims. Indeed, Myles had a history of supporting the Irish Volunteers. Shortly before the outbreak of the First World War, Myles agreed to use his private yacht, the *Chotah*, to transport guns to Ireland for the Irish Volunteers.[112] Despite his distinguished service in the RAMC during the war, he continued his support for the IRA during the War of Independence and utilised his position as surgeon in the Richmond Hospital to secure the appropriate treatment for the IRA's wounded while at the same time, shielding them from arrest. In 1919, the IRA brought Matt Brady, a junior IRA officer who was severely wounded in a tussle with two members of the Royal Irish Constabulary in County Longford, to the Richmond Hospital. He was treated by Thomas Myles, who locked Brady 'into presses and other places of concealment when the place was being searched by Black and Tans and other British forces'.[113] Michael O'Dea, an Irish volunteer wounded during the Easter Rising, also recalled that he remained in hospital for three weeks under Myles' care, who, he said, 'did not allow any of the wounded to fall into British hands'.[114]

During the Irish Civil War, demobbed RAMC medical personnel had the opportunity to continue their army work in the newly formed Irish National Army. Established in January 1922, it was the official army of the Irish Free State. Under the temporary guidance of Commandant-General Ahern, the National Army Medical Corps for the new army was created a month later. The medical corps initially consisted of those who had had connections with the separatist nationalists prior to 1920. Brigade MOs from the IRA formed a skeleton service and approximately 300 non-commissioned officers and men, without previous military experience or training, joined the corps. For the most part, jobs in the medical corps appealed to newly qualified medical personnel who had struggled to secure employment elsewhere or establish profitable private practices. Remuneration in the National Army Medical Corps was much lower than in general practice and few doctors in private practice were prepared to lose income and enlist.[115]

Following the outbreak of the Irish Civil War in June 1922, the National Army expanded in size and ex-British Army servicemen enlisted in numbers. Leonard has estimated that ex-British servicemen accounted for approximately half of the 55,000 in the National Army.[116] In August 1922, the National Army Medical Corps was expanded and reorganised. Due to the high number of casualties in County Cork, Ahern travelled there to take charge and Maurice Hayes was subsequently appointed as head of the National Army Medical Corps.[117] Hayes utilised his First World War experience with the IMWC and recruited additional doctors for the corps, including many RAMC veterans. Bernard Forde, who had served with No. 6 Clearing Hospital in France during the Great War and had held the rank of Lieutenant Colonel in the RAMC, was appointed alongside Hayes to the Irish Army Medical Council. Francis Morrin, a UCD graduate who had served with the RAMC in France and aboard the *Mauretania* hospital ship, was appointed as surgeon and Officer in Charge at the Curragh Hospital, which was part of the National Army's medical infrastructure and catered for many of its casualties.[118] At its wartime maximum, the National Army Medical Corps comprised 110 whole-time MOs, 200 part-time MOs and 500 NCOs, two whole-time senior surgeons, two senior consultants and a changing number of junior surgeons.[119] In 1925, Peter Hughes, Minister for Defence for the

Government of the Irish Free State, acknowledged that this had been a large force but that during the Civil War, 'the Army medical service had a very large amount of work to do. Our posts were small and scattered, and it naturally took more doctors to see that the men got proper treatment than it would in normal times'.[120] Many of these doctors had participated in the First World War as members of the RAMC.[121]

To assist Hayes' search for medical personnel during the Civil War, the National Army increased the budget for the medical corps. In February 1923, the army introduced a new salary structure for MOs (Table 5.2).

In April 1923, an article in the *British Medical Journal* stated that 'it is understood that when the end of the present civil war is reached the necessity for the present comparatively large service will cease'.[122] This was not entirely accurate—while some MOs demobilised from the medical corps following the end of the conflict, many continued. By 1925, there were still 543 personnel in the National Army Medical Corps, including 85 MOs who were on year-to-year contracts. In defence of the number of MOs still attached to the Corps, Hughes argued in a Dáil Éireann debate that

> while some salaries, as they appear on the estimate, may appear alarming, if we are to get the right class of men for the service we must pay them well. We have had a number of resignations on account of the small pay that some of the men were getting. As a matter of fact, during the past six months some of our best men have resigned.[123]

**Table 5.2**  Salaries for medical officers of the Irish National Army Medical Corps, 1923

| Position | £ | s. | d. | |
|---|---|---|---|---|
| Lieutenant | 1 | 0 | 0 | Per day |
| Captain | 1 | 10 | 0 | Per day |
| Commandant | 2 | 2 | 0 | Per day |
| Colonel | 1000 | 0 | 0 | Per annum |
| Deputy Director | 1250 | 0 | 0 | Per annum |
| Major-general | 1500 | 0 | 0 | Per annum |

*Source* Anon., 'Free State Army Medical Service' in *British Medical Journal*, 3249, no. 1 (1923), p. 609

Major Bryan Cooper TD, who had served in the First World War with the Connaught Rangers, criticised the expenditure on the medical corps:

> the British have one man in the Medical Corps to every forty in the army and we have one to every thirty-five. That ought to be corrected ... the British army is serving all over the world in all sorts of climates and conditions. Its units extend from Hong Kong to Jamaica, and we, surely, in this matter of medical services, ought to be able to administer our affairs more cheaply and better, and more efficiently, because the men are all serving in their own country. They have no violent extremes of climate.[124]

Due to the criticism from Cooper and others, the number of MOs attached to the National Army Medical Corps soon dwindled with recruitment restricted. As a result, long-term service in the National Army Medical Corps was not a viable option for the majority of Ireland's RAMC veterans and by 1925, they had to look elsewhere for suitable employment.

## CONCLUSION

This chapter has argued that the First World War adversely affected the Irish medical profession. While the war initially relieved the pressure on an overcrowded profession, ultimately, it was only a temporary reprieve. Medical demobilisation, elongated and complex, was poorly managed. The War Office's decision to, at first, slowly release doctors back into civilian medical infrastructure and then, to later, initiate extensive demobilisation ensured that civilian medical services experienced an initial dearth and then a surfeit of doctors. Although it has been demonstrated that RAMC veterans pursued several alternative career options, a considerable number of doctors demobilised from the British Army returned to Ireland. Consequently, in the 1920s, the Irish medical profession was once again severely overcrowded demonstrating that the conflict significantly escalated the pre-war congestion of the Irish medical profession identified by Jones.[125] It is thus contended that enlistment in the RAMC was an impediment to career development for many Irish doctors. While doctors who held government or hospital posts before the war returned to their pre-war occupations, newly qualified doctors who had enlisted directly into the British Army medical services after graduation struggled to secure employment in Ireland's overcrowded profession. For some general practitioners, their practices were interrupted or lost and thus they were forced to look elsewhere for employment. In Ireland, the LGBI's stubborn refusal to lift the wartime employment veto following the signing of the Armistice coupled with the outbreak of influenza placed the medical profession under significant pressure. This indicates that the LGBI failed to grasp that the poor law medical services required additional doctors to cope with the increased workload that was perpetuated by influenza. Given the relationship between guardians and the LGBI during this period, it is likely that the LGBI's refusal also signified their desire to assert authority over Ireland's poor law guardians. Disagreements between the LGBI and guardians regarding medical appointments in the aftermath of war were thus part of a wider political battle in Ireland.

RAMC doctors also returned to a volatile Ireland, which would soon be in the midst of domestic warfare. Fitzpatrick and Leonard have shown that returning British Army soldiers were subject to a hostile reaction.[126] It has been posited here that returning doctors sometimes experienced difficulty in securing positions as a consequence of their ties to the British Army. However, in other cases, the IRA ultimately coveted army doctors for their professional skill and wartime experience.

## NOTES

1. Dr. A. C. Pearson, *Hull Daily Mail*, 20 November 1920.
2. Ross McKibbin, 'Great Britain' in Robert Gerwarth (ed.), *Twisted paths: Europe, 1914–45* (Oxford: Oxford University Press, 2007), p. 39.
3. Ackroyd et al., *Advancing with the army*, p. 217.
4. Adam Seipp, *The ordeal of peace: Demobilization and the urban experience in Britain and Germany, 1917–21* (London: Routledge, 2009), p. 44.
5. For more on demobilisation of combatants, see Stephen Richards Graubard, 'Military demobilization in Great Britain following the First World War' in *The Journal of Modern History*, 19, no. 4 (1947), pp. 297–311; Seipp, *The ordeal of peace*, pp. 47–90.
6. Fitzpatrick, *Politics and Irish life*, p. 168; Jane Leonard, 'Survivors' in Horne (ed.), *Our war*, pp. 211–231.
7. Daly, *The buffer state*, p. 47.
8. Daly, *The buffer state*, p. 48.
9. Donnacha Seán Lucey, *The end of the Irish poor law? Welfare and health-care reform in revolutionary and independent Ireland* (Manchester: Manchester University Press, 2015), p. 19.

10. Lucey, *The end of the Irish poor law?* p. 5.
11. Daly, *The buffer state*, p. 29.
12. For more on local government in Northern Ireland, see Alvin Jackson, 'Local government in Northern Ireland, 1920–73' in Mary E. Daly (ed.), *County and town: One hundred years of local government in Ireland* (Dublin: Institute of Public Administration, 2001), pp. 56–66.
13. Jackson, 'Local government in Northern Ireland', p. 60.
14. Anon., 'Medical demobilisation' in *Supplement to the British Medical Journal*, 3028, no. 1 (1919), p. 53.
15. Michael Mahoney (RCPI, Kirkpatrick Index, TPCK/5/3).
16. Black, *King's nurse*, p. 125.
17. Letter from Frank C. Eve to the editor in *British Medical Journal*, 3026, no. 2 (1918), p. 731.
18. Letter from Herbert Butcher to the editor in *British Medical Journal*, 3027, no. 1 (1919), p. 28.
19. *Irish Independent*, 9 January 1919.
20. Anon., 'The Central Medical War Committee and medical demobilization' in *British Medical Journal*, 3031, no. 1 (1919), p. 134.
21. Anon., 'The Irish Medical War Committee' in *British Medical Journal*, 3044, no. 1 (1919), p. 560.
22. *Irish Independent*, 18 June 1918.
23. Abraham, *Surgeon's journey*, p. 247.
24. Seipp, *The ordeal of peace*, p. 163.
25. Anne Rasmussen, 'The Spanish flu' in Winter (ed.), *The Cambridge history of the First World War: Civil society*, p. 335.
26. Foley, *The last Irish plague*, p. 3.
27. Foley, *The last Irish plague*, p. 25. Also see Patricia Marsh, 'The war and influenza: The impact of the First World War on the 1918–19 influenza pandemic in Ulster' in Durnin and Miller (eds.), *Medicine, health and Irish experiences of conflict, 1914–45*, pp. 31–44.
28. *Irish Independent*, 7 December 1918.
29. Foley, *The last Irish plague*, p. 35; Ida Milne, *Stacking the coffins: Influenza, war and revolution in Ireland, 1918–19* (Manchester: Manchester University Press, 2018); Marsh, 'The war and influenza', pp. 31–44.
30. Foley, *The last Irish plague*, p. 35.
31. *Freeman's Journal*, 26 October 1918.
32. *Freeman's Journal*, 26 October 1918.
33. *Anglo-Celt*, 14 December 1918.
34. *Westmeath Examiner*, 18 January 1919.
35. *Westmeath Examiner*, 21 June 1919.
36. *Kildare Observer*, 20 December 1920.

37. *Belfast Newsletter*, 30 December 1918.
38. Veto discussed in Chapter 2.
39. Ida Milne, 'Influenza: The Irish Local Government Board's last great crisis' in Lucey and Crossman (eds.), *Healthcare in Ireland and Britain from 1850*, p. 233.
40. *Limerick Leader*, 9 January 1919.
41. *Limerick Leader*, 9 January 1919; the Castletown Board of Guardians were traditionally a radical board. See William L. Feingold, 'The tenant's movement to capture the Irish Poor Law Boards, 1877–1886' in *Albion: A Quarterly Journal Concerned with British Studies*, 7, no. 3 (1975), p. 227.
42. *Irish Independent*, 11 January 1918.
43. *Kildare Observer*, 22 March 1919.
44. Of course, Irish doctors had returned from temporary commissions throughout the war years but their return was most evident following the large demobilisation in April 1919.
45. Black, *King's nurse*, p. 129.
46. Benson, 'The effect of war on the medical profession', p. 94.
47. Francis Crosbie (RCPI, Kirkpatrick Index, TPCK/5/3).
48. John Green (RCPI, Kirkpatrick Index, TPCK/5/3).
49. Other examples include Samuel Elgee who secured a post in a mental hospital in Cane Hill, Surrey; Alfred Elliott who established a private practice in Nottingham; George Culverwell took up a position as a school medical officer for Berkshire County Council; Frederick Clarke, who had a private practice in Tyrone prior to the war secured the house surgeon post in the Royal Infirmary, Sheffield. Sources: RCPI, Kirkpatrick Index, TPCK/5/3; *British Medical Journal*, 1917–1935.
50. Abraham, *Surgeon's journey*, p. 247. Abraham was not the only doctor to give up their private practices while enlisted in the army medical services. Several others, including Lewis Crowe, an Irish doctor with a private practice in Chester, closed his practice in 1915 so he could serve with the RAMC. For more, see RCPI, Kirkpatrick Index, TPCK/5/3.
51. Abraham, *Surgeon's journey*, p. 248.
52. Abraham, *Surgeon's journey*, p. 248.
53. Whitehead, *Doctors in the Great War*, p. 258.
54. *Irish Times*, 12 August 1966.
55. Meyer, *Men of war*, p. 97.
56. *First and second special reports from the Select Committee on Pensions together with the proceedings of the committee and minutes of evidence and appendices* [Cd. 247], H.C. 1919, vi, 138. For more on the Ministry of Pensions in Ireland, see Michael Robinson, '"Nobody's children?": The Ministry of pensions and the treatment of disabled Great War veterans

in the Irish Free State, 1921–1939' in *Irish Studies Review*, 25, no. 3, pp. 316–335.

57. *Irish Times*, 31 May 1918.

58. *First and second special reports from the Select Committee on Pensions together with the proceedings of the committee and minutes of evidence and Appendices* [Cd. 247], H.C. 1919, vi, 181.

59. Bourke, *Dismembering the male*, p. 89.

60. Bourke, *Dismembering the male*, p. 90.

61. *First and second special reports from the Select Committee on Pensions together with the proceedings of the committee and minutes of evidence and Appendices* [Cd. 247], H.C. 1919, vi, 447.

62. Anon., 'Dr. Harold Saunderson sugars' in *British Medical Journal*, 3567, no. 1 (1929), p. 935.

63. Ackroyd et al., *Advancing with the army*, p. 224.

64. Whitehead, *Doctors in the Great War*, p. 256.

65. *Belfast Newsletter*, 28 March 1919.

66. Cooter, 'Medicine and the goodness of war', pp. 147–159.

67. Abraham, *Surgeon's journey*, p. 251.

68. Anon., 'Shortage of doctors' in *British Medical Journal*, 3054, no. 2 (1919), p. 64.

69. *Irish Independent*, 10 April 1919.

70. *Drogheda Independent*, 26 April 1919.

71. *The Liberator*, 3 May 1919.

72. Kelly, *Irish women in medicine*, pp. 135–158.

73. Kelly, *Irish women in medicine*, pp. 135–158.

74. *Irish Times*, 14 September 1922.

75. Anon., 'Ireland' in *British Medical Journal*, 3011, no. 2 (1918), p. 299; *Donegal News*, 12 October 1918; *Irish Times*, 25 September 1919.

76. *Weekly Freeman's Journal*, 2 March 1918.

77. *Nenagh Guardian*, 20 December 1919.

78. *Nationalist and Leinster Times*, 28 February 1920.

79. Anon., 'Shortage of doctors' in *British Medical Journal*, 3054, no. 2 (1919), p. 64.

80. *Annual report of the Local Government Board for Ireland, for the year ended 31st March, 1919, being the forty-seventh report under the Local Government Board (Ireland) Act, 1872* [Cmd. 578] H.C. 1920, xxvii.

81. *Dublin Evening Telegraph*, 24 March 1920.

82. *Irish Times*, 11 March 1920.

83. *Irish Times*, 11 March 1920.

84. *Irish Independent*, 15 March 1920.

85. As discussed in David Durnin, 'Ireland's British Army doctors and the treatment of Irish nationalists, 1916–23' in David Durnin and Ian

Miller (eds.), *Medicine, health and Irish experiences of conflict, 1914–45* (Manchester: Manchester University Press, 2017), pp. 94–108.

86. *First and second special reports from the Select Committee on Pensions together with the proceedings of the committee and minutes of evidence and Appendices* [Cd. 247], H.C. 1919, vi, 443.

87. Jane Leonard, 'Facing the finger of scorn: Veterans' memories of Ireland after the Great War' in Martin Evans and Ken Lunn (eds.), *War and memory in the twentieth century* (Oxford: Berg, 1997), p. 59.

88. Fitzpatrick, *Politics and Irish life*, p. 136.

89. Abraham, *Surgeon's journey*, p. 248.

90. Leonard, 'Getting them at last', p. 118.

91. E. O'Halpin, 'Problematic killing during the war of independence and its aftermath: Civilian spies and informers' in J. Kelly and M. A. Lyons (eds.), *Death and dying in Ireland, Britain and Europe: Historical perspectives* (Kildare: Irish Academic Press, 2013), p. 332.

92. Paul Taylor, *Heroes or traitors? Experiences of Southern Irish soldiers returning from the Great War, 1919–1939* (Liverpool: Liverpool University Press, 2015), pp. 243–244.

93. *Hull Daily Mail*, 20 November 1920.

94. William Murphy, *Political imprisonment and the Irish, 1912–21* (Oxford: Oxford University Press, 2014), p. 100.

95. Taylor, *Heroes or traitors?* p. 250.

96. *Belfast Newsletter*, 6 August 1920.

97. Letter from Dr. Richard Hennessy, presented at the National Library of Ireland collection day organised by Europeana 1914–18, a project which brings together resources from three major European projects each dealing with different types of First World War material. Accessed at http://www.europeana1914-1918.eu/fr/contributions/3418, 12 March 2014 (hereafter Europeana).

98. Letter from Dr. Richard Hennessy (Europeana, 1914–18 collection).

99. *Irish Independent*, 20 May 1931.

100. *Irish Examiner*, 7 November 1919.

101. *Irish Examiner*, 7 November 1919.

102. *Irish Examiner*, 17 May 1919.

103. *Irish Examiner*, 17 May 1919.

104. *Nationalist and Leinster Times*, 20 December 1919.

105. *Nationalist and Leinster Times*, 18 September 1920.

106. Anon., 'Ireland', *British Medical Journal*, 28 April 1923, p. 148.

107. Anon., 'Ireland', *British Medical Journal*, 30 April 1921, p. 136.

108. Anon., 'Ireland', *British Medical Journal*, 24 April 1920, p. 125.

109. As detailed in Durnin, 'Ireland's British Army doctors', pp. 100–103.

110. A similar situation had unfolded in nineteenth-century Ireland. Barry Kennerk has argued that army doctors who had experience in dealing with gunshot wounds from their participation in wars elsewhere treated the wounded of the Irish Republican Brotherhood as a consequence of their wartime expertise. See Barry Kennerk, 'In danger and distress: Presentation of gunshot cases to Dublin Hospitals during the height of Fenianism, 1866–71' in *Social History of Medicine*, 24, no. 3 (2011), pp. 588–607.
111. Witness statement of William O'Hora (BMH, collection of witness statements, WS1554), p. 15.
112. Witness statement of Sean Fitzgibbon (BMH, collection of witness statements, WS30); Durnin, 'Ireland's British Army doctors', p. 102.
113. Witness statement of Sean MacEoin (BMH, collection of witness statements, WS1716).
114. Witness statement of Michael O'Dea (BMH, collection of witness statements, WS1152).
115. *Freemans Journal*, 13 August 1923; Durnin, 'Ireland's British Army doctors', p. 102.
116. Leonard, 'Survivors', p. 219.
117. Outbreaks of violence were rife in County Cork during the Civil War. See Peter Hart, *The I.R.A. and its enemies: Violence and community in Cork, 1916–23* (Oxford: Oxford University Press, 1998).
118. *Irish Times*, 13 July 1968.
119. Duggan, *A history of the Irish Army*, p. 109.
120. Peter Hughes, *Dáil Éireann debates*, 14 May 1925.
121. *Freemans Journal*, 13 August 1923.
122. Anon., 'Free State Army Medical Service' in *British Medical Journal*, 3249, no. 1 (1923), p. 609.
123. Peter Hughes, *Dáil Éireann debates*, 14 May 1925.
124. Major Bryan Cooper, *Dáil Éireann debates*, 14 May 1925.
125. Jones, 'Strike out boldly'.
126. Fitzpatrick, *Politics and Irish life*, p. 136.

# CHAPTER 6

# The Impact of the First World War on Irish Hospitals, 1918–1925

'The Government had problems to settle to-day which left the problems of the hospitals in the shade'.[1]

There was little change in the hospital arrangements for sick and wounded soldiers who returned for treatment in Ireland in the period immediately after the Armistice. It was not until 1919 that the War Office sought to reduce expenditure on medical services and instructed the RAMC to decrease the number of beds reserved for soldiers in hospitals in Ireland and Britain. In November 1918, there were approximately 364,000 hospital beds reserved for sick and wounded soldiers in military, specialist and civilian hospitals throughout Britain and Ireland. This was the highest number of beds reserved at any time during the conflict. However, beginning in January 1919, this figure fell rapidly as the War Office relinquished their claims to beds in civilian institutions and smaller military hospitals began to close. MacPherson has estimated that by November 1919, the number of military beds still in use was approximately 50,000.[2]

Leonard has estimated that about 100,000 war veterans returned to Ireland between November 1918 and the summer of 1920.[3] Among them were injured men who required hospital treatment and consequently, a number of specialist hospitals and war wards remained open to provide medical care. Some of the smaller military hospitals had closed before the Armistice because they were costly and inefficient. As early as

© The Author(s) 2019
D. Durnin, *The Irish Medical Profession and the First World War*,
Medicine and Biomedical Sciences in Modern History,
https://doi.org/10.1007/978-3-030-17959-5_6

November 1916, Lloyd George, at a debate in the House of Commons, had argued that the minor military hospitals in Omagh, County Tyrone; Enniskillen, County Fermanagh and Dundalk, County Louth were unsuitable for the reception of the returning sick and wounded, and were a drain on government finances. Consequently, these institutions closed.[4] This chapter will focus on the restructuring of hospital services for ex-servicemen in the years after the Armistice—1918 to 1925. It will examine both specialist and civilian hospitals and assess the effect of changing military policies on these institutions. As shown, the war had generated new income streams for Ireland's civilian hospitals and increased revenue significantly. Ultimately, by 1918, the financial position of hospitals deteriorated due to spiralling rates of inflation that negatively affected most Irish medical institutions. The chapter will examine the financial state of Ireland's civilian hospitals after the end of hostilities assessing whether these institutions recovered throughout the 1920s.

Following the outbreak of the Irish War of Independence in 1919 and the Irish Civil War in 1922, hospital governors had additional difficulties to overcome to ensure that their hospitals continued to admit patients. A detailed historiography of the conflicts and the tension in the years preceding them has built up in recent years.[5] No study, however, has considered the impact of the civil disturbance on the country's medical infrastructure. This chapter will explore the considerable difficulties that arose for hospitals as a result of the domestic war and examine the problems these institutions faced in caring for both the ex-First World War serviceman and those from the IRA.

## POST-WAR RECONSTRUCTION OF MILITARY MEDICAL CARE

Following the Armistice, the responsibility for organising medical treatment for wartime soldiers gradually shifted from the War Office to the MOP. The War Office covered the cost of treatment of those still in the British Army, while the MOP financed the medical care of ex-servicemen. As an increasing number of soldiers were demobilised from the army, the MOP became primarily responsible for organising medical treatment for the majority of those who had fought in the First World War. Only soldiers in receipt of pensions were entitled to treatment at the expense of the MOP. In July 1919, an Army Council instruction detailed the process through which ex-servicemen in need of medical care in military hospitals secured assistance:

discharged soldiers applying for treatment in a military hospital should, in the first instance, be referred to the War Pensions Committee, from whom a formal application for admission will be received, if the man is found to be eligible for treatment. Military hospitals will not admit discharged soldiers unless application has been made by the Ministry of Pensions or by a War Pensions Committee.[6]

While numerous new hospitals opened in Ireland during the First World War to treat soldiers, there was a considerable reduction in medical facilities for military cases—soldiers and ex-soldiers—following the Armistice. By the summer of 1919, the British Red Cross and others began to close the hospitals that they had established in Ireland for the treatment of soldiers. Cooter's study of orthopaedics in the First World War has indicated that the medical benefits of war did not necessarily extend beyond the war years.[7] This thesis can be applied to hospital provision for soldiers. Following the Armistice, hospital provision for soldiers in Ireland, for the most part, quickly reverted to its pre-war state. Smaller Red Cross hospitals soon began to close. In June 1919, the Red Cross formally closed the twenty-four bed Dublin University Auxiliary Hospital which was located at Mountjoy Square. Established in the home of Mr and Mrs Picton Bradshaw, who provided their house free of rent to the Red Cross, it had admitted shell-shock sufferers from February 1915 until its closure.[8] Almost a week later, the Dublin Castle Red Cross Hospital closed having treated 6946 patients since opening at the beginning of 1915.[9] Other hospitals, outside of the control of the Red Cross and established solely for the purposes of treating soldiers, also closed. In the winter of 1919, the asylum governors at both the Belfast War Hospital and the Richmond War Hospital at Grangegorman closed their wards for soldiers.[10]

Soldiers in these institutions were consequently transferred to civilian hospitals and this put pressure on the civilian medical infrastructure. Bourke has argued that war exacerbated the problem of the shortage in accommodation for disabled civilians in Britain, as the war-maimed soldiers were sent to facilities that had been intended for civilian use.[11] Evidently, this was also the case in Ireland.[12] In December 1919, following the announcement that the Richmond War Ward was to close, the asylum governors transferred twenty-seven ex-servicemen within the month to other civilian asylums, including those in Limerick and Derry.[13] The movement of soldiers into beds intended for civilian use decreased the number of beds available for non-military patients and put pressure on already overcrowded institutions.

Due to the reduction in the number of beds available in military hospitals, ex-soldiers entered poor law hospitals. Poor law guardians admitted them and retrospectively claimed payment from the MOP. In March 1920, the Ballyshannon Board of Guardians, County Donegal, met to discuss the costs associated with treating ex-British Army soldiers.[14] Usually, poor law guardians recruited specialist doctors on an ad hoc basis to operate on ex-soldiers in the union hospital. Some guardians expressed concerns about the costs associated with this work—approximately one guinea per operation—and argued that 'the Government should bear the expense'.[15] Dr. Walsh, a local dispensary doctor and speaking as a medical referee, informed the guardians that they could send the patients to other hospitals and the MOP would still cover the cost. He claimed that 'there was any amount of money for the treatment of these ex-soldiers, and the ratepayers should not suffer in any way'.[16] In this instance, the guardians secured payment from the MOP to cover the cost of the operations in their own hospital.

By 1920, multiple boards of guardians stopped admitting ex-British Army soldiers into the workhouse hospitals. In July 1920, the Ballyshannon guardians refused to admit any soldiers into their workhouse hospital and Dr. McCarthy, an LGBI inspector, argued that the guardian's decision excluded the men simply 'because they had served in the army'.[17] In response, the guardians maintained that 'the British Government should look after these ex-soldiers and provide hospital treatment for them. We refuse to take them in. This hospital was and is maintained for the sick and poor of the district and not for ex-army men'.[18] Subsequently, the LGBI dropped the matter.[19] It is likely that the guardians' decision to stop admitting the soldiers was part of the wider hostility towards the LGBI.

Given the closure of the Red Cross hospitals and the increasing hostility of poor law guardians, the MOP maintained their own hospitals in Ireland in the years after the war. Before the signing of the Armistice, the MOP, surely aware that the hospitals opened for military cases during conflict would ultimately close, had begun to expand medical infrastructure for soldiers and established their own hospitals in Ireland to treat specialist cases and this included ex-soldiers suffering from neurasthenia.[20] In July 1917, Lieutenant Colonel James Craig offered his house and large grounds in Craigavon, County Armagh, to the UVF

Hospital Board of Management to be used as a neurasthenic hospital and this eventually came under the control of the MOP.[21] In September 1917, the ministry secured another mansion and estate in Leopardstown Park, Dublin, from Lady Talbot Power, for the purposes of providing treatment to neurasthenic soldiers. Opened in 1918, the hospital had accommodation for 136 ex-servicemen suffering from paralysis, loss of speech and loss of hearing or sight.[22] In 1920, the Ministry took control of the other specialist hospital operating under its aegis—the surgical and orthopaedic hospital for disabled soldiers in Blackrock, County Dublin.

These hospitals remained open into the 1920s and beyond and continued to treat ex-soldiers. Yet the accommodation in these hospitals was insufficient for the number of soldiers who required treatment in Ireland. Bourke has suggested that southern Ireland had the highest proportion of ex-servicemen awaiting treatment for neurasthenia in the United Kingdom.[23] In 1921, representatives from the MOP in Ireland requested funding from the central MOP board to expand facilities but they were refused due to its desire to cut costs.[24] Therefore, while MOP hospitals became increasingly important to the medical care of ex-servicemen in 1920s Ireland due to the closure of other hospitals, ultimately, they were unable to treat all soldiers who required treatment. Instead, the MOP focused on continuing its relationship with Ireland's network of civilian hospitals.

## CIVILIAN HOSPITALS

Adopting the War Office's earlier strategy, the MOP rented beds in existing Irish hospitals, north and south, to accommodate soldiers. These arrangements with civilian hospitals had been in place since the closing stages of the conflict. By late 1918, hospitals provided beds to both the War Office and the MOP. In October, for instance, the War Office requested the governors of the Meath Hospital in Dublin to provide extra accommodation for soldiers from the expeditionary forces. On the same date, the MOP also submitted a request for the provision of beds for ex-soldiers. The governors of the Meath Hospital set aside number seven ward, containing twenty-three beds for military use—allocating fifteen for the expeditionary forces and eight beds for the MOP sponsored patients.[25]

**Table 6.1**   Income from War Office and MOP to the Dublin House of Industry Hospitals, 1920–1925

| Income source | 1920–1921 | 1921–1922 | 1922–1923 | 1923–1924 | 1924–1925 |
|---|---|---|---|---|---|
| War Office | £262,130 | £84,435 | £19,250 | £0 | £0 |
| Ministry of Pensions | £21,309 | £22,162 | £20,669 | £9822 | £8662 |

*Source* Board of Superintendence of the Dublin Hospitals Annual Reports, 1920–1925

Ireland's civilian hospitals had suffered financial hardship during the war and this continued in the decade after the Armistice. Initially, however, the hospitals benefited from several streams of income and donations associated with the end of the war, including income from the War Office and MOP. In 1920–1921, voluntary hospitals in England and Wales had an income of approximately £2 million and about a quarter of this came from MOP funds, provided to cover the cost of military patients.[26] In Ireland, this income stream constituted an even larger proportion of revenue for some hospitals. In the 1920–1921 financial year, forty-seven per cent of the Dublin House of Industry Hospitals' total income came from the War Office and MOP (Table 6.1).

Civilian hospitals also benefited from donations presented to them for their war work and in memory of soldiers and medical personnel who died in the war. The Royal Victoria Hospital in Belfast received several donations following the end of the war including a donation of 1400 francs on behalf of Lieutenant–General Sir Beauvois de Lisle of the 15th Corps in 'recognition of the many valuable services rendered by the staff of the hospital to soldiers and their dependents during the war'.[27] From 1918 onwards, committees were established in towns throughout Ireland to generate funds for war memorials. Banks and businesses, including Leinster Bank and the Guinness Brewery, erected memorials to employees and former students who had been killed in the war.[28] Doctors and medical students paid for memorials and endowed beds in hospitals in memory of their former colleagues. In 1920, Sir Patrick Dun's Hospital, Dublin, unveiled a memorial bed and tablet in honour of thirty past students of the hospital 'who laid down their lives in the Great War'.[29] Similarly, families sponsored beds as memorials to their relatives in Dublin hospitals at a cost of £50 per bed, per year.[30] In October 1918, the Royal City of Dublin Hospital received £500 from the Moore

Memorial Fund to endow a bed indefinitely in memory of those who fought in the First World War on condition it be occupied by members of the various branches of the British Army.[31]

The closure of Red Cross branches and hospitals across the country also brought benefits to the civilian hospitals. The British Red Cross raised and spent approximately £21 million in Britain and Ireland during the war; a significant proportion equipped domestic hospitals.[32] As well as utilising funds from the central committee, the Red Cross in the three southern provinces of Ireland raised at least £500,000 over the course of the conflict.[33] As the Red Cross wards and hospitals began to close, the society transferred some of its assets to civilian hospitals. As the 1920 Official War Report of the British Red Cross in Ireland explained: 'during the year following the Armistice, the work of the Joint War Committee seemed to increase rather than diminish and the demobilisation of the various hospitals and numerous Red Cross organisations entailed heavy work'.[34] At the time of its closure, the Dublin University Hospital had a balance of £328 that had been raised from the sale of the institution's furniture and this money was donated to Sir Patrick Dun's Hospital.[35] Similarly, on 5 May 1919, the County Wexford Branch of the British Red Cross Society informed the governors of several Dublin hospitals that the Wexford branch of the society was shutting down and that they intended to donate the remaining cash to the civilian hospitals. The Society wanted to reserve one bed for Wexford convalescent soldiers and their dependants who required treatment and offered £400 to several hospitals to cover the costs.[36] In Northern Ireland, the Royal Ulster Joint VAD Committee—British Red Cross Society and SJA—donated larger sums to a smaller number of hospitals from funds that it had raised during the war. In one of its most sizeable contributions of the immediate post-war years, the committee donated £10,000 to the Royal Victoria Hospital in March 1920.[37] In total, Abel-Smith assessed that hospitals throughout Britain and Ireland received approximately £1,360,000 from the surplus war funds of the British Red Cross Society.[38] Tables 6.2 and 6.3 provides details a sample of Irish hospitals that received funds and demonstrates how the Red Cross' different approach to fund dispersal in Ulster and the rest of Ireland influenced the amount contributed to each hospital.

Following the closure of wartime hospitals, there was a considerable number of spare beds and equipment no longer needed and the voluntary organisations donated some of this to the civilian hospitals.

**Table 6.2**  Sample of Dublin hospitals that received funds from the Red Cross during demobilisation

| Hospital | £ | s. | d. |
|---|---|---|---|
| Stillorgan Convalescent Home | 100 | 0 | 0 |
| Royal City of Dublin | 109 | 11 | 9 |
| Peamount Sanatorium | 350 | 1 | 0 |
| Adelaide | 81 | 9 | 3 |
| Mater, Dublin | 81 | 9 | 3 |
| Meath | 137 | 7 | 0 |
| Mercer's | 81 | 9 | 4 |
| St. Vincent's | 81 | 9 | 3 |
| Richmond | 81 | 9 | 3 |
| Dr. Steevens' | 81 | 9 | 3 |
| Jervis Street | 81 | 9 | 3 |
| Sir Patrick Dun's | 81 | 9 | 3 |
| Monkstown | 56 | 7 | 3 |

*Source Red Cross in Ireland*, p. 32

**Table 6.3**  Sample of Ulster hospitals that received funds from the Red Cross during demobilisation

| Hospital | £ | s. | d. |
|---|---|---|---|
| Hilden Convalescent Hospital, Belfast | 9500 | 0 | 0 |
| Mater Infirmorum Hospital | 3000 | 0 | 0 |
| Royal Victoria Hospital | 10,000 | 0 | 0 |
| UVF Hospital | 5000 | 0 | 0 |

*Source Northern Whig*, 5 May 1925

For example, Major T. Houston informed the board of management of the Royal Victoria Hospital in Belfast that the SJA intended to offer a large amount of equipment to the hospital's pathological laboratory. The equipment was from a hospital in France where Houston had been working.[39] Similarly, on the day of its closure, the Board of the Dublin Red Cross Hospital offered its beds and equipment to hospitals and local educational institutions—they presented a complete x-ray apparatus to the RCSI and approximately £400 worth of supplies to Jervis Street and Sir Patrick Duns hospitals.[40]

Irish hospitals also benefitted from the Red Cross and SJA's post-war reorganisation of war hospital supply depots. During the conflict, the Red Cross and SJA, along with other voluntary groups, had organised a network of war hospital supply depots throughout Ireland. The Red Cross and SJA's central depot was housed at 40 Merrion Square in Dublin and an additional eight sub-depots were situated in various locations throughout the country. Over the course of the war, approximately 6500 women worked in the depots supplying dressings to hospitals in Britain, Egypt, France, India, Ireland, Salonika and elsewhere.[41] In the immediate aftermath of the conflict, the smaller depots gradually closed with their supplies and funds often transferred to local hospitals. The Joint War Committee of the British Red Cross and SJA in Ireland decided to continue the work of the central supply depot for the benefit of civilian hospitals and to: 'take their share in tackling the many health problems of a civilian character in the country as well as aiding the discharged soldier now under the Ministry of Pensions'.[42] Subsequently, the committee retained the *c.* £70,000 collected by the 'Our Day' organisation in 1918 and renewed their lease on the property at Merrion Square for ten years, where it set up its headquarters. Dorothy Hignett, Deputy Head of the Irish War Hospital Supply Depot, further detailed the reasoning behind the decision:

> Having a very good quantity of the finest surgical material which had been purchased at an exceedingly advantageous rate, the committee feel that if this could be used to make surgical supplies it would be the means of helping the civilian hospitals to purchase their dressings at reasonable terms.[43]

Hospital governors supported the proposal and in November 1919, the Irish Hospital Supply Depot, a successor to the Irish War Hospital Supply Depot, opened at 51 Lower Mount Street, Dublin.[44] Over 50,000 items were distributed to hospitals the following year.[45] In 1920, the Red Cross declared that in the supply depots' focus on national health, women were the 'leaders and pioneers'.[46]

Despite benefitting in several different ways from the end of the war, in the longer term the conflict and its subsequent aftermath had a negative impact on Ireland's civilian hospitals. These institutions were perilously close to complete collapse in the decade after the war. Even with the significant income derived from the MOP and voluntary bodies, hospitals could not balance the accounts. In 1918, the outbreak of influenza further undermined hospital finances. Hospital governors in several institutions were forced to pay additional salaries to doctors and nurses drafted into replace and assist regular staff members during the influenza outbreaks.[47] As medical personnel succumbed to the disease, staff numbers in several institutions dropped considerably. On 28 October 1918, the governors of the Meath Hospital reported that 'owing to the present epidemic, the acting house surgeon and four of the staff sisters are laid aside sick' and the hospital was severely short staffed. A hospital nurse, nurse Dulig, died from the disease.[48] Dispensary MOs were put under significant pressure; Dr. Byrne, MO, Grand Canal Street dispensary, Dublin, requested that the Dublin guardians provide him with an assistant to cope with the increasing workload due to the influenza outbreak. When this request was denied, he complained that

> He has 27 years' service and never before asked for assistance, and did not do so until he found it was impossible for any one medical man to attend all the cases ... unless this epidemic subsides it would be utterly impossible for any one medical man to attend to the sick cases which require attention.[49]

Hospital salary budgets spiralled out of control in the years after the war. While this can be attributed partly to increasing staffing levels, it was primarily the result of post-wartime inflation. In Britain, the inflationary trend generated by wartime conditions continued for a number of years and this damaged the hospital system.[50] The same was true in Ireland. By 1923 the salaries of the nursing staff at the Meath Hospital amounted to more than the hospital's entire expenditure in 1913.[51] In July 1919, the Lord Mayor of Dublin, Laurence O'Neill, announced at a corporation meeting that the Richmond, Whitworth and Hardwicke Hospitals would have to close that month if additional funds could not be found.[52] While the hospitals did not completely close—admissions were limited for a time—the situation highlighted their severe financial difficulties. They also lacked government support and the board repeatedly urged the government to increase its grant to the hospitals.

A government grant of £7600 had been awarded annually to several Dublin hospitals though the rate had not changed since it was first introduced in 1855. Despite requests from the hospital governors during the war, the Treasury refused to increase the amount.[53] Barrington Jellet, chairman of the board of governors of the House of Industry

Hospitals, criticised the government's refusal as 'a callous cruel thing, which showed there was something very rotten in the administration'.[54] On 29 January 1920, Dr. Edward Coey Bigger, Crown Representative for Ireland on the British General Medical Council, in a memorandum to the Irish Public Health Council—appointed by the Chief Secretary for Ireland in 1919 to formulate proposals on an Irish public health bill— claimed that 'unless some means of rendering financial assistance can be found many of the hospitals will have to restrict their operations, and in some cases may have to close down altogether'.[55] Coey Bigger explained that a number of potential solutions had been examined but that 'there is no likelihood of the state taking over these hospitals, nor would it be desirable to abolish the system of voluntary control, and some other means must be found of providing additional funds'.[56]

Responding in June 1920, Dublin's hospital governors attended a public meeting held in the lecture theatre of the Royal Dublin Society to discuss the financial difficulties of eleven of Dublin's hospitals, including the Adelaide, Dr. Steevens' Hospital and the House of Industry Hospitals.[57] The gathering intended to highlight the disastrous financial position of the hospitals and initiate a scheme to raise approximately £100,000 to alleviate the debts of Dublin's hospitals. In his address to the meeting, Lord Powerscourt stated that

> he thought he was right in saying that nothing had ever been attempted before on such a scale in Dublin – to raise £100,000 to pay off the debts on practically all the hospitals, but they were not deterred in the slightest degree by the prospect ... he had not the slightest doubt they would reach their ultimate goal ... this was the people's last piece of clearing up in Dublin after the war.[58]

He called upon the city's population to replicate the generosity they had shown during the war. The committee's plans to raise the money centred on various fund-raising initiatives including appeals and fetes, which hospitals had run repeatedly in the previous decades.[59]

The attempt would ultimately end in failure. Raising such a large amount of money was not an easy task as public charitable donations to Ireland's hospitals declined in the years after the war. While post-war unemployment did not peak in Ireland until the 1930s, the war destabilised the global economy and encouraged economic disruption and chronic depression, which impacted on charitable donations.[60]

Barry Supple argues that this atmosphere was not unique to the First World War but it attained crippling levels of intensity in the early twentieth century.[61] In addition, the breakdown of governance in Ireland exacerbated the country's economic difficulties. During the early 1920s, arrears in local authority rates mounted as a consequence of the breakdown in the system of tax collection. As Daly posits, there was little prospect of local authorities providing additional resources for hospitals.[62] Likewise, due to the depression, businesses and the public were unable or reluctant to continue giving the hospitals financial support. At the 1923 annual meeting of the Meath Hospital, the secretary bemoaned that 'bad trade and unemployment had affected the contributions from employers and employees alike, while heavy taxation and the state of the country rendered it impossible for many subscribers to continue their support'.[63]

In addition, a considerable number of hospital subscribers cancelled their donations following the armistice feeling that they had 'done their bit'. As Abel-Smith has perceptively argued, 'wounded soldiers made excellent appeal copy and the purse-strings of the charitable public were unloosened as they have perhaps never been before'.[64] During the war, the public were very aware of the need to support the treatment of soldiers through charitable activities, as the number of casualties mounted and large numbers of wounded were transported through towns to hospitals.[65] However, the presence of wounded soldiers still in receipt of treatment in civilian hospitals in the 1920s was not as well publicised and subscriptions declined. Moreover, there is a correlation between the end of the regular dockings of hospital ships and the highly publicised unloading of troops, and the decline in subscription rates. As early as Christmas 1918, there were already signs in Ireland that public interest in the well-being of soldiers was declining. On 14 December 1918, a letter from an anonymous contributor, published in the *Kildare Observer*, urged readers to continue to support soldiers in hospitals:

> the hospitals are still full of the men who have helped to make this peace a glad reality for us at Firmount Hospital there are forty men. Would it not be a good idea to let our thank offerings [sic] take the form of gifts to make their Christmas a happy one? By this time last year there was a long list of gifts promised; this year there are only three promised. Surely we shall not allow our peace Christmas to fall below the standard of our war one?[66]

Martin Gorsky and John Mohan have found that by 1921, sixty-eight per cent of London's hospitals were in debt, with a total deficit at nearly £400,000; for many this meant the need to increase borrowing.[67] In Britain, hospitals' financial well-being soon began to improve as legacies, gifts and interest on previous endowments to hospitals increased in value.[68] A similar trend was evident in the financial accounts of the larger hospitals in Ulster. In 1922, the treasurer of the Royal Victoria Hospital in Belfast reported that the hospitals debt had reduced from £6830 to £463 due to donations from generous contributors and an increase in investments.[69] The hospital also benefitted from its increasingly generous workplace subscription list, which had become instrumental to the hospital's financial security during the war. The workplace subscriptions soared into the 1920s—in 1905, the subscription list amounted to £5076 but by 1923, it had grown to £19,155 and it was the hospital's leading source of income by 1925.[70]

In contrast, the finances of hospitals elsewhere in Ireland continued to deteriorate as subscriptions declined even further. At a meeting in 1921, the Cork Joint Hospital and Labour Committee sought to raise funds to ease 'the alarming debt resting on the local hospitals'.[71] John Lumsden, in his role as Vice-Chairman of the Joint War Committee of the British Red Cross and SJA, informed the public that when the headquarters in London requested co-operation for another effort to raise money for the Red Cross, his committee refused; 'as we feel strongly that at the present time every effort of this character should be directed towards the collection of funds for the hospitals, which are so sadly in need of assistance'.[72] Table 6.4 charts the decreasing amounts of subscriptions and donations for several of Dublin's civilian hospitals, including Steeven's, Meath and House of Industry hospitals.

Civil unrest was partly responsible for declining hospital subscriptions in Ireland. Due to the War of Independence and Civil War, wealthy

**Table 6.4**  Income from subscriptions and donations for Dublin civilian hospitals, 1920–1925

|  | 1920–1921 | 1921–1922 | 1922–1923 | 1923–1924 | 1924–1925 |
|---|---|---|---|---|---|
| Subscriptions and donations | £13,667 | £16,402 | £11,639 | £8717 | £8592 |

*Source* Board of Superintendence of the Dublin Hospitals Annual Reports, 1920–1925

Protestant philanthropists, who were among the hospitals' largest contributors, had departed Ireland in the early 1920s. In 1921, the Lord Chancellor of Ireland, Sir John Ross, addressed the annual meeting of Sir Patrick Dun's Hospital Linen Guild in Dublin. Ross acknowledged the financial difficulties facing the hospitals and argued that

> owing to the disturbed state of the country, a great number of those who formerly were our best supporters are leaving the country. I am sorry for that. I think everybody should stand his ground. But still the fact remains that they are going ... Ireland is being impoverished of these good people, and England and Scotland are getting them.[73]

Similarly, the Board of the Victoria Hospital, Cork, argued at their 1923 annual general meeting that their £321 fall in income from subscriptions, donations and collections was primarily due to the 'departure from Ireland of so many of our subscribers'.[74]

In England, Scotland and Wales, the voluntary hospitals were assisted by a significant parliamentary grant of £500,000 paid from the treasury in 1921, which was to be distributed among the institutions to help eliminate their debts. The provision of a one-off grant to hospitals was a solution proposed by a special parliamentary committee, chaired by Viscount Cave, which was established to solve the voluntary hospitals' financial problems that arose due to war. Published in 1921, Cave's report recommended exemptions from tax on gifts and donations and a temporary treasury grant to rescue the hospitals from the immediate crisis.[75] Yet Irish hospitals were deemed not to be entitled to it. Cave's report noted that Irish hospitals, north and south, were 'not included in our reference'.[76] Sir Henry McLaughlin, one of Ireland's prominent builders and developers, criticised the British government for refusing to extend the voluntary hospital grant to Ireland because the finance was distributed to help hospitals to 'overcome a difficulty created by the government themselves through the late war ... the debt was almost entirely a war debt'.[77] In defence of the decision, the Chief Secretary stated that Ireland now 'had a parliament of its own'.[78] Hospital governors thus requested members of the Dáil to consider increasing the funding for the hospitals.

In June 1920, the Dáil established a Commission on Local Government to examine potential reforms and cost-cutting measures. Many of the savings proposed were from the health sector. These included a reduction of £25,000 in funding for services for venereal

disease and child welfare schemes; £50,000 saved through the aboli-
tion and amalgamation of workhouses; £10,000 from a reduction in the
number of patients with tuberculosis undergoing hospital treatment; and
the amalgamation of hospitals.[79] Eventually, in 1924, the newly created
Department of Local Government and Public Health assumed control
of responsibilities for public medical services from the LGBI and implemented a number of these cost-saving plans. For example, poor law
unions and boards of guardians were dissolved and replaced by boards
of public assistance and health.[80] These reforms were the first attempt
to dismantle the poor law in either Great Britain or Ireland.[81] Although
the new department was aware of the problems that blighted the hospital
system, it did little to alleviate them and ultimately, ignored voluntary
hospitals.[82] In June 1923, Ernest Blythe, Minister for Local Government
of the Free State, admitted that 'the past few years had been very hard
on these voluntary hospitals but this was not the time to rush into proposals that might put a very serious charge on the State'.[83]

Due to the significant fall in income, increased expenditure and the
Irish government's refusal to increase grants, voluntary hospital governors were forced to re-evaluate their approach to financing healthcare. Gorsky and Mohan have argued that hospital administrators in
Britain conceded that traditional charitable sources could not provide
long-term stability, given the extension of personal taxation during the
war.[84] Hospital governors and local authorities in Ireland had a similar outlook on the matter. In March 1921, the Lord Chancellor, Sir
James Campbell, reported to the Committee of the Dublin Associated
Hospitals Fund that changes had been made in the administration of the
hospitals in Dublin that he 'hoped would relieve the public to a large
extent of the perpetual appeals for assistance'.[85] The initiatives included
increasing income from local authorities. Campbell noted that 'county
councils would bear a fair share of the expenses incurred by the hospitals in treating the inhabitants of their districts'.[86] In addition, hospitals
were increasing income from paying-patients. A similar shift was occurring in Britain at this time. By 1920, nearly all hospitals in London were
charging patients.[87] Before the war, the income from paying patients in
six Dublin hospitals, including the Meath and the Mater, averaged at
£2000 a year but by the 1920s it had risen to £24,000.[88] Several public
representatives criticised the hospitals for this approach and argued that
paying patients received treatment before the poor but ultimately, the
hospital governors argued that they had little choice.[89]

Despite the increase in income from paying patients, finances in most Irish hospitals continued to deteriorate in post-war Ireland. Expenses also continued to soar. Wages in several hospitals increased as new medical staff were hired to care for ex-soldiers and existing medical staff sought additional payments on the basis that the hospitals were receiving additional money from the MOP for admitting veterans. When the medical staff of the Royal Victoria Hospital in Belfast considered whether they were well-equipped to care for MOP patients, they deemed it necessary for the hospital governors to hire an additional house surgeon with two pupils as well as the visiting staff that were already in situ.[90] On 25 March 1918, the board of governors of the Meath Hospital had agreed to 'allot to the medical staff 5s. weekly for each soldier treated in the wards'.[91] On 8 April 1920, Sir John Moore, a governor of the Meath Hospital, criticised his fellow board members for failing to fulfil their promise to pay hospital medical staff, arguing that no payments had been made to the medical staff since the initial one. The board concurred and reaffirmed that 5s. a week would be paid to the medical and surgical staff for attendance on discharged soldiers.[92] In addition, the Honorary Secretary of the Medical Board requested that the governors set aside twenty-five per cent of fees paid by the MOP for treatment to extern ex-soldiers, who were treated outside of the hospital wards, to be allocated to the MOs attending such patients. The governors unanimously agreed.[93]

The rise in paying patients entering the wards also brought problems. Daly has argued that the wealthier, middle-class patients sought high-quality medical care from hospitals equipped with the latest advances in medical technology.[94] This was one of several factors that encouraged some of Ireland's hospitals, in difficult financial circumstances, to increase expenditure on equipment. New departments were formed. One of the most popular additions to hospitals was an x-ray department. In the early twentieth century, many hospitals adopted radiotherapy.[95] During the war, x-rays had become a staple of medical treatment and the departments became the central hub of hospital radiology.[96] In 1924, Mercer's Hospital installed a new x-ray machine, which increased the work of the hospital's radiology department. In addition, several hospitals purchased sun lamps, used to deliver UV light to patients with skin diseases.[97] Due to the considerable advances in medical equipment, hospital expenditure continued to rise. In 1925, the head of x-ray department in Mercer's warned the governors that, despite the purchase of the new machine:

It is not to be concluded that no further expenditure upon this department will be necessary for many years. Manufacturers of x-ray equipment are making rapid strides in the elaboration and perfecting of apparatus, and almost every month that passes sees the introduction of some new appliance which becomes necessary ... Within the past year a new hot-Cathode X-ray tube has been introduced, and has just come upon the market, and is a tremendous advance upon all previous models. The hospital has just ordered one of these and expects delivery within the next few days. It is hardly necessary to remind the public that a department of this kind cannot be maintained in a state of maximum efficiency without their continued generous support.[98]

By the 1920s, as well as requiring upgrades of equipment, many hospitals were badly in need of structural improvements. In 1924, the Board of Sir Patrick Dun's Hospital appealed for £100,000 to rebuild the institution. The board informed the public that

repeated efforts had been made to alter and improve some of the arrangements of the hospital, but the main fabric of the building remains substantially as it existed one hundred and twenty years ago, and, after careful investigation, it has been found impossible to alter it to meet modern requirements except at a prohibitive cost and with a questionable result.[99]

Needless to say, the hospital failed to raise £100,000 for the project.

With increased expenditure and insufficient income streams, the majority of Irish civilian hospitals plunged further into debt and hospital authorities continued to blame the First World War for financial difficulties. In 1924, A. G. Hollinshead, Honorary Treasurer for the Royal Hospital for Incurables, Dublin, published a letter in the *Irish Times* to 'call the attention of a generous and sympathetic public to the merits and urgent needs of one of our greatest and most deserving charities, the Royal Hospital for Incurables'.[100] The hospital had accommodation for approximately 250 patients; however, similar to other Irish hospitals, it was suffering from severe financial difficulties. According to Hollinshead, 'having suffered from the effects of the late world war, it finds itself in debt to the bank in upwards of £9000'.[101] Even the Royal Victoria Hospital in Belfast, despite its impressive income, recorded a debt of approximately £500 for 1924.[102]

A change in the MOP's policy caused further difficulty for hospital governors and adversely affected several hospitals that had previously benefited from MOP income. According to the secretary of the Meath Hospital, the Ministry had decided 'that it was more economical and more convenient to send ex-servicemen for treatment to two or three of the larger hospitals'.[103] Consequently, the Dublin House of Industry Hospitals—the Richmond, Hardwicke and Whitworth—received the vast majority of MOP patients and income. Other hospitals, which had previously been in receipt of this income, suffered; for example, the income the Meath Hospital received from the MOP fell from £3470 in 1922 to £993 in 1923 and ceased altogether in 1925.[104] Similarly, in Northern Ireland the Ulster Joint Committee of the British Red Cross and SJA had attempted to keep the Hilden Convalescent Hospital for ex-servicemen, located in Belfast, open but the MOP declined their offer. Instead, the MOP decided that one hospital was sufficient and they 'opted to keep the UVF Hospital running'.[105] The UVF Hospital Committee consequently purchased the Hilden Red Cross Hospital for £8000 and used the buildings to treat ex-servicemen.[106]

Given the declining levels of income and increasing costs, it can be persuasively argued that Ireland's voluntary hospitals suffered financially as a consequence of the First World War. Increasing levels of inflation, perpetuated by wartime conditions, ultimately endangered the Irish hospital network and this threat did not cease with the signing of the Armistice. While financial difficulty was certainly hospital governors' main cause for concern, other issues also arose in 1920s Ireland, which were detrimental to the workings of the hospitals.

## THE IMPACT OF CONFLICT IN IRELAND ON HOSPITALS, 1919–1923

As well as dealing with financial problems, Ireland's hospital governors had to cope with additional difficulties associated with treating ex-British soldiers in revolutionary Ireland. Disabled British Army soldiers in civilian hospitals were often targets of sectarian threats. In February 1922, Catholic ex-soldiers in Craigavon Disabled Soldiers Hospital in Belfast received threats from anonymous sources warning them to leave the hospital. Approximately half of the fifty patients in Craigavon Hospital were Catholics. A letter received by one Catholic ex-serviceman warned him to leave before the week was out:

you are the oldest R.C. in there, and all the others are known; so look out what you get if any of you traitor dogs are got about the place in 3 days from now. Death to rebels and papists, red hand for ever. Don't blame men in hospital, but we won't have you among loyalists. You low bred swine. You and your sieeking [sic] dogs of Papish – must go. £5 reward won't save yous, nor will Popes, Priests, Holy Water ... Time's up. Go or we will riddle every rotten Papish both in Craigavon and U.V.F., as you are a rotten lot of Bastards'.[107]

Colonel W. B. Spender, Secretary to the Cabinet, Northern Parliament, remarked in a letter to Lionel Curtis, adviser to the colonial secretary on Irish affairs, that:

I regret to say that I am afraid there has been intimidation of Roman Catholic ex-servicemen in this hospital, both by anonymous correspondence and in at least one case by personal threats addressed to patients. The hospital authorities have done everything in their power to safeguard their Roman Catholic patients and probably the threats are not really of a very serious character – from purely a physical point of view – but when conveyed to ex-servicemen suffering from shell-shock, they are of the most cowardly character and unfortunately produce great effect on the individual ... I also hear that at least one threat has recently been given to Protestant ex-servicemen at this institution but this is no doubt, merely a reprisal.[108]

The Catholic ex-servicemen were transferred to another hospital following receipt of this telegraph.[109] Their new location was not published in the press.

Moreover, medical staff in the hospitals had to cope with additional security concerns due to conflict in their locality. In Belfast, the Superioress of the Mater Hospital, Belfast, wrote to the President of the International Red Cross in June 1922 to inform him of shots fired at the hospital:

the police are easily excited and shoot indiscriminately left and right. During the night of the 5th instant, between 11pm and 12 midnight, we were suddenly subjected to a veritable siege lasting 45 minutes, the said constabulary shooting against our hospital with machine guns. What I ask of you Mr President is that the rules of the Red Cross may be applied to us here and that we be afforded protection from attacks of this nature, because during the war your society always maintained that hospitals should be respected by all combatants. We have confidence in the forces of the British Empire and we should desire to be protected by them.[110]

The hospital authorities reported that 'serious material damage was done to the building and patients were terrorised by gunfire lasting over forty-five minutes. Several of the patients, medical staff and nurses had narrow escapes from bullets which swept the wards ... it is almost incredible that such an atrocity could be perpetrated on a hospital'.[111] Sir Robert Kennedy, County Director of Belfast and Director in Chief for Ulster British Red Cross and Order of St. John, was informed by Colonel Spender that the firing was due to suspicions that some of the young medical students actually fired from the hospital buildings. Spender noted that 'on the night before the particular attack was made, the police reported that there was a sniping post on the hospital, and there are special reasons for not making this fact public'.[112] Hospital staff strongly denied this accusation and the damage to the hospital was repaired. The incident demonstrated that hospital staff and administrators in Ireland not only had to cope with the damaging aftermath of the First World War, but also with the problems involved in providing healthcare in the midst of violent domestic conflict.

Other incidents, which left hospital medical staff fearful, were reported throughout Ireland. In December 1922, John McArdle, surgeon at St. Vincent's Hospital, Dublin, emphasised the security fears of hospital staff in Ireland in a letter published in the *British Medical Journal*. McArdle detailed an event during which members of the IRA attempted to rescue a comrade who was undergoing treatment in Mercer's Hospital. On this occasion, the military policeman in charge of the hospital was shot.[113] McArdle complained that

until now we surgeons thought our hospitals were refuges sacred from interference. During the Black and Tan regime Irish surgeons were commanded ... to notify the authorities of the reception of the wounded ... I am happy to say Irish surgeons gave no report. During all this time there was no instance of an attack made in hospitals by any member of the army of occupation. It is with extreme regret I learned this morning that an unprecedented occurrence at Mercer's Hospital demonstrated that parties, unthinking of the well-being of Ireland, discredited one of the sanctuaries of the people of Ireland by an attempted murder ... I desire to enter a protest against the invasion of these sanctuaries, which have always afforded a willing, beneficent, and unselfish devotion to all, regardless of status, who required their aid.[114]

McArdle mentioned the passing of a military order, issued in 1921 by crown forces, which caused considerable unrest among Irish hospital staffs. It required doctors to 'furnish daily particulars of wounded persons under their care in hospital', essentially acting as informants for the crown forces.[115] On 10 January 1921, the Colonel Commandant of Dublin District wrote to the staff at Stevens' hospital:

[I] order you, the Secretary, being the person in charge of Doctor Stevens Hospital to furnish to me in writing the names and descriptions of all persons admitted to your hospital who are or are suspected to be suffering from wounds caused by bullets, gun fire or other explosives together with such particulars and information concerning them as may be within your knowledge. Such information is to be furnished by you daily ... failure to comply with this order will render you liable to proceeded against for an offence against the restoration of order in Ireland regulations.[116]

Several anonymous fellows, licentiates and other Irish medical personnel sent letters to the Council of the RCSI requesting that they intervene and ask the military to revoke the order, arguing that it would be a 'breach of professional confidence'.[117] In response, the military insisted that failure to comply with the Order would render the medical practitioners liable under the Restoration of Order in Ireland Regulations.[118] The IRA issued their own warning, and threatened hospital medical staff who obeyed the military order that they 'would be treated as spies'.[119] Sir William Wheeler, Vice-President of the RCSI Council, issued a copy of the council's response to the Irish Medical Secretary:

the Council are of opinion that it is contrary to the public interest that medical men should break their professional tradition and, without the consent of their patients, disclose information which they have obtained in the discharge of their professional duties. If any instance is reported to the council in which one of the fellows or licentiates of the College is pressed to break confidence, such specific case will be considered by the Council, and representations made to the authorities if such be thought necessary.[120]

The Council also proclaimed that in the event of medical personnel carrying out the order, 'wounded members of the Irish republican army would be disposed rather to die from their wounds than seek medical aid when doing so meant for a certainty their trial at a later date by the military authority'.[121] It is difficult to ascertain whether any hospital staff complied with the military order, but given the level of opposition towards it, and the public backing the RCSI Council gave those who ignored it; it is unlikely that many adhered to it. However, the threats made the hospital wards a tense working environment for hospital staff in the post-world war period.

As well as disturbing the daily workings of the civilian hospitals, the change in Ireland's relationship with Britain also altered the administrative structures managing Ireland's military hospital network. Following the signing of the Anglo-Irish Treaty, the British Army transferred the remaining major military hospitals, located in the Irish Free State, to the control of the Irish National Army. In 1923, the Irish Army Medical Service had taken control of the King George V Hospital, which had been the centre of British Army medical administration in Ireland, and renamed it as St. Bricin's Hospital.[122] Similarly, the Irish Army Medical Service assumed control of the Curragh Hospital. Peter Hughes, Minister for Defence, argued that it was essential to retain Ireland's military hospitals as 'soldiers must be kept under discipline when they are sick as well as when they are well. It is not possible to send a number of soldiers to a private hospital and leave them without the discipline they would be under when receiving treatment in a military hospital'.[123]

Members of the Dáil debated whether these military hospitals were required due to the high cost. Major Bryan Cooper criticised Hughes' reasoning regarding discipline, and argued that

> I have been a patient in an army hospital and in a civilian hospital, and I can assure the Minister that the discipline is the same in both places, and that the mildest hospital nurse that was ever born is a more rigid martinet than the most severe disciplinarian in the Army. Any patient in any hospital is at the mercy of the authorities, because when they take away your trousers you are helpless, and they invariably do.[124]

Cooper suggested that soldiers be admitted to civilian hospitals instead with the cost of their care covered by the government. This suggestion was supported by Sir James Craig, who had been physician to the Lord Lieutenant of Ireland prior to entering politics as an MP and later TD for Dublin University. Craig posited that considering the 'diminution in the strength of the army, and the disappearance of fighting and therefore of wounds, and that ... the amount of illness should be small in a young and healthy army, the work could be very easily undertaken by the general hospitals in Dublin and Cork'.[125] Despite Cooper and Craig's arguments, St. Bricin's and the Curragh Military Hospital remained in operation and these institutions, which had been integral to British Army's casualty evacuation programme in Ireland during the First World War, became central components of the Irish Free State's military medical infrastructure.

## CONCLUSION

This chapter has considered the long-term impact of war on Ireland's civilian—voluntary and some state—hospital system. The outcomes of the war—inflation, a weak economy and influenza—combined to seriously threaten the existence of Irish civilian hospitals. In the years immediately after war, hospital governors sought potential solutions. Such was the scale of the crisis, in 1924 the governors of Sir Patrick Dun's proposed an amalgamation of five Dublin hospitals—the Meath, the Adelaide, Mercer's, Sir Patrick Dun's and the Royal City of Dublin. The governors at Dun's hospital campaigned for funds for the construction of a new central Dublin hospital which would replace the five smaller institutions. While the proposal was not successful—the governors failed to secure the funding and the idea was abandoned three years later—the incident demonstrates the scale of the problem.[126] Other initiatives were subsequently implemented to try and improve the situation, culminating in the introduction of the hospitals sweepstake—a lottery established in the Irish Free State in 1930 to fund the hospitals.[127] It was not until the 1930s, following the introduction of the Irish hospitals' sweepstake, that hospitals began to show an element of financial stability. The sweepstake continued to fund Irish hospitals for over fifty years. Therefore, the war pushed the Irish civilian hospital system to unprecedented levels of financial instability and possible closure, encouraging those in charge of hospital finance continued to seek new ways of funding their hospitals.

## NOTES

1. *Freemans Journal*, 1 June 1920.
2. MacPherson, *History of the Great War*, p. 94.
3. Leonard, 'Survivors' in Horne (ed.), *Our war*, p. 211.
4. *Irish Times*, 11 November 1916.
5. Fitzpatrick, *Politics and Irish life*; Bill Kissane, *The politics of the Irish War* (Oxford: Oxford University Press, 2005); Anne Dolan, *Commemorating the Irish Civil War: History and memory, 1923–2000* (Cambridge: Cambridge University Press, 2006); For more on Irish Civil War, see Fitzpatrick, *Revolution?*; Michael Hopkinson, *Green against green: The Irish Civil War* (Dublin: Gill and Macmillan, 2004); Edward Purdon, *The Irish Civil War, 1922–23* (Cork: Mercier Press, 2000).
6. *Irish Times*, 12 July 1919.
7. Cooter, *Surgery and society*, p. 105.
8. *Irish Times*, 7 June 1919.
9. *Irish Independent*, 18 May 1921.
10. Dawson, 'The work of the Belfast War Hospital', p. 16.
11. Bourke, *Dismembering the male*, p. 49.
12. *Freemans Journal*, 22 September 1922.
13. Admission and discharge book for the Richmond War Hospital (NAI, uncatalogued).
14. Boards of Guardians in County Donegal were traditionally dominated by a radical majority, which tended to become nationalist strongholds. See Feingold, 'The tenants' movement to capture the Irish Poor Law boards, 1877–86', p. 227.
15. *Fermanagh Herald*, 6 March 1920.
16. *Fermanagh Herald*, 6 March 1920.
17. *Fermanagh Herald*, 17 July 1920.
18. *Fermanagh Herald*, 17 July 1920.
19. *Fermanagh Herald*, 17 July 1920.
20. Bourke, 'Effeminacy, ethnicity and the end of trauma', p. 66.
21. Anon., 'Craigavon neurasthenic hospital for soldiers, Belfast' in *British Medical Journal*, 2952, no. 2 (1917), p. 132; Bourke, 'Effeminacy, ethnicity and the end of trauma', p. 66.
22. For more on this hospital, see Eoin Kinsella, *Leopardstown Park Hospital 1917–2017: A home for wounded soldiers* (Dublin: Leopardstown Park Hospital, 2017).
23. Bourke, 'Effeminacy, ethnicity and the end of trauma', p. 66.
24. Bourke, 'Effeminacy, ethnicity and the end of trauma', p. 67.
25. Meath Hospital minute book, 14 October 1918 (NAI, NAI/2007/128).
26. Abel-Smith, *The hospitals*, p. 295.

27. *Belfast Newsletter*, 18 September 1919.
28. Leonard, 'Lest we forget', p. 60.
29. *Irish Times*, 9 December 1920.
30. *Irish Times*, 9 December 1920.
31. Royal City of Dublin Hospital minute book, 8 November 1918 (NAI, 2006/98).
32. Abel-Smith, *The hospitals*, p. 255.
33. Order of St. John, *The Red Cross in Ireland*, p. 11.
34. Order of St. John, *The Red Cross in Ireland*, p. 30.
35. *Irish Times*, 7 June 1919.
36. Meath Hospital minute book, 5 May 1919 (NAI, NAI/2007/128).
37. Management committee book for Royal Victoria Hospital, 3 March 1920 (PRONI, MIC/514/1/1/21).
38. Abel-Smith, *The hospitals*, p. 324.
39. Anon., 'Royal Victoria Hospital, Belfast' in *British Medical Journal*, 3033, no. 1 (1919), p. 199.
40. *Royal College of Surgeons in Ireland seventy-seventh annual report—year ending 5th April, 1920*, 1920 (RCSI, uncatalogued); *Irish Independent*, 18 September 1919.
41. Margaret Downes, 'The civilian voluntary aid effort' in Fitzpatrick (ed.), *Ireland and the First World War*, p. 35.
42. Order of St. John, *The Red Cross in Ireland*, p. 30.
43. Meath Hospital minute book, 14 October 1918 (NAI, NAI/2007/128).
44. Order of St. John, *The Red Cross in Ireland*, p. 31.
45. *Irish Times*, 11 December 1920.
46. Order of St. John, *The Red Cross in Ireland*, p. 17.
47. Abel-Smith, *The hospitals*, p. 278.
48. Meath Hospital minute book, 28 October 1918 (NAI, NAI/2007/128).
49. South Dublin Union Board of Guardians' minute book, 9 July 1918 (NAI, MFGS 49/91).
50. Abel-Smith, *The hospitals*, p. 295.
51. Anon., 'Meath Hospital, Dublin' in *British Medical Journal*, 3258, no. 1 (1923), p. 993.
52. *Freemans' Journal*, 22 February 1919.
53. Hospitals in receipt of government grant—Westmoreland Lock, Steevens' Hospital, Meath Hospital, Cork Street Hospital, House of Industry Hospitals (Richmond, Hardwicke, Whitworth), Rotunda Lying-in Hospital, Coombe Lying-in Hospital, Royal Victoria Eye and Ear Hospital, Royal Hospital for Incurables.
54. Anon., 'Dublin hospitals' in *British Medical Journal*, 3059, no. 2 (1919), p. 218.

55. *Irish Times*, 29 January 1920.
56. *Irish Times*, 29 January 1920.
57. The other hospitals were the Meath, Mercer's, Royal City of Dublin, Sir Patrick Dun's, the Coombe, the Rotunda, Cork Street Fever Hospital and the National Eye and Ear Hospital.
58. *Freemans Journal*, 1 June 1920.
59. *Freemans Journal*, 1 June 1920.
60. Kitchen, *Europe between the wars*, p. 76.
61. Barry Supple, 'War economies' in Winter (ed.), *The Cambridge history of the First World War. The state*, p. 295.
62. Daly, 'An atmosphere of sturdy independence: The state and the Dublin hospitals in the 1930s' in Jones and Malcolm (eds.), *Medicine, disease and the state in Ireland*, p. 237.
63. Anon., 'Meath Hospital, Dublin' in *British Medical Journal*, 3258, no. 1 (1923), p. 993.
64. Abel-Smith, *The hospitals*, p. 282.
65. Winter, 'Hospitals', p. 358.
66. Letter from Anon to the editor, *Kildare Observer*, 14 December 1918.
67. Martin Gorsky, John Mohan and Tim Willis, *Mutualism and health care: British hospital contributory schemes in the twentieth century* (Manchester: Manchester University Press, 2006), p. 33.
68. Abel-Smith, *The hospitals*, p. 323.
69. *Belfast Newsletter*, 31 March 1922.
70. *Belfast Newsletter*, 12 June 1924; *Belfast Newsletter*, 26 March 1926.
71. *Irish Examiner*, 8 December 1921.
72. *Irish Times*, 25 October 1920.
73. Anon., 'Loss to Irish hospitals' in *British Medical Journal*, 3176, no. 2 (1921), p. 813.
74. *Irish Examiner*, 19 March 1923.
75. Gorsky et al., *Mutualism and health care*, p. 33.
76. *Ministry of Health, Voluntary Hospitals Committee. Final Report* [Cmd. 1335] H.C. 1921, XIII.
77. *Irish Independent*, 27 June 1921.
78. Anon., 'Loss to Irish hospitals' in *British Medical Journal*, 3176, no. 2 (1921), p. 813.
79. Daly, 'An atmosphere of sturdy independence', p. 238.
80. Sean Lucey, '"These schemes will win for themselves the confidence of the people": Irish independence, poor law reform and hospital provision' in *Medical History* 58, no. 1 (2014), p. 51.
81. Lucey, 'These schemes will win for themselves the confidence of the people', p. 52; In Northern Ireland, the poor law system was retained until 1939.

82. Daly, 'An atmosphere of sturdy independence', p. 237.
83. Anon., 'Hospital grants and public health legislation' in *British Medical Journal*, 3258, no. 1 (1923), p. 993.
84. Gorsky et al., *Mutualism and health care*, p. 34.
85. Anon., 'Ireland' in *British Medical Journal*, 3142, no. 1 (1921), p. 439.
86. Anon., 'Ireland' in *British Medical Journal*, 3142, no. 1 (1921), p. 439.
87. Abel-Smith, *The hospitals*, p. 297.
88. Barrington, *Health, medicine and politics in Ireland*, p. 108.
89. Barrington, *Health, medicine and politics in Ireland*, p. 108.
90. Medical Staff Minute Book for the Royal Victoria Hospital, Belfast, 10 October 1918 (PRONI, MIC514/1/2/3).
91. Meath Hospital minute book, 12 April 1920 (NAI, NAI/2007/128).
92. Meath Hospital minute book, 12 April 1920 (NAI, NAI/2007/128).
93. Meath Hospital minute book, 12 April 1920 (NAI, NAI/2007/128).
94. Daly, 'An atmosphere of sturdy independence', p. 238.
95. Stevens, *Medical practice in modern England*, p. 38.
96. Christopher Lawrence, 'Continuity in crisis: Medicine, 1914–45' in W.F. Bynum, Anne Hardy, Stephen Jacyna, Christopher Lawrence, E.M. Tansey (eds.), *The western medical tradition, 1800 to 2000* (Cambridge: Cambridge University Press, 2006), p. 270.
97. Lawrence, 'Continuity in Crisis', p. 274; For more on light therapy see Tania Anne Woloshyn, *Soaking up the rays: Light therapy and visual culture in Britain, c. 1890–1940* (Manchester: Manchester University Press, 2017).
98. *Mercer's* Hospital, *Dublin: Report for 1925* (Dublin, 1926), p. 33.
99. Anon., 'Sir Patrick Dun's Hospital' in *British Medical Journal*, 3322, no. 2 (1924), p. 388.
100. *Irish Times*, 14 April 1924.
101. *Irish Times*, 14 April 1924.
102. *Belfast Newsletter*, 25 March 1925.
103. Anon., 'Meath Hospital, Dublin' in *British Medical Journal*, 3258, no. 1 (1923), p. 993.
104. *Board of Superintendence of the Dublin Hospitals reports*, 1922–1925.
105. *Belfast Newsletter*, 4 May 1925.
106. *Belfast Newsletter*, 4 May 1925.
107. *Freemans Journal*, 27 February 1922.
108. Letter from Colonel W.B. Spender, D.S.O., M.C.; Secretary to the Cabinet, Northern Parliament, to Lionel Curtis, Colonial Office, 'Craigavon Hospital: Intimidation of Catholic ex-servicemen' Public Record Office of Northern Ireland, 24 March 1922 (PRONI, CAB/6/9).
109. *Freemans Journal*, 27 February 1922.

110. Letter from Sister Molda to the President of the International Red Cross, 9 June 1922 (PRONI, CAB/6/47).
111. *The Scotsman*, 7 June 1922.
112. Letter from Colonel Spender to Robert Kennedy, 20 June 1922 (PRONI, CAB/6/47).
113. Surgeon McArdle, 'Hospitals as sanctuaries' in *British Medical Journal*, 3234, no. 2 (1922), p. 1248.
114. Surgeon McArdle, 'Hospitals as sanctuaries' in *British Medical Journal*, 3234, no. 2 (1922), p. 1248.
115. Anon., 'Reports on wounded in Dublin Hospitals' in *British Medical Journal*, 3234, no. 1 (1921), p. 319.
116. Colonel Commandant, Dublin District, to the Secretary, Dr. Steevens' Hospital, Dublin, 10 January 1921 (RCPI, Dublin Clinical Hospitals Committee minute book, DCHC/5).
117. Anon., 'Reports on wounded in Dublin Hospitals' in *British Medical Journal*, 3139, no. 1 (1921), p. 319.
118. Anon., 'Reports on wounded in Dublin Hospitals' in *British Medical Journal*, 3139, no. 1 (1921), p. 319.
119. Anon., 'Reports on wounded in Dublin Hospitals' in *British Medical Journal*, 3139, no. 1 (1921), p. 319.
120. Anon., 'Wounded in Hospital' in *British Medical Journal*, 3143, no. 1 (1921), p. 477.
121. Anon., 'Wounded in Hospital' in *British Medical Journal*, 3143, no. 1 (1921), p. 477.
122. *Freeman's Journal*, 8 January 1923.
123. Peter Hughes, *Dáil Éireann debates*, 14 May 1925.
124. Major Bryan Cooper, *Dáil Éireann debates*, 14 May 1925.
125. James Craig, *Dáil Éireann debates*, 14 May 1925.
126. Coleman, *The Irish sweep*, p. 11.
127. Coleman, *The Irish sweep*, pp. 1–15.

CHAPTER 7

# Conclusions

Between 1914 and 1925, the Irish medical profession experienced extensive disruption and alteration. The First World War occurred in the context of increasing political division and rising nationalist sentiment in
Ireland. In the course of these events, members of the Irish medical profession enlisted into the British Army to serve in the war. A key concern
of this study has been to analyse the enlistment trends of Irish doctors
into the British Army during the conflict. Callan and Fitzpatrick have
suggested that in the early months of the war, Irish men—non-medical—
joined the British Army in large numbers but enlistment figures fell
around the midpoint of the conflict before rising again in 1918.[1]
Meanwhile, Whitehead has argued that doctors in Britain also enthusi-
astically enlisted into the British Army medical services, until the number
of available medics was exhausted.[2] It has emerged in this study that Irish
doctors enlisted in a pattern comparable to doctors in Britain, rather
than their fellow countrymen entering the combat forces. Like their
British counterparts, Irish doctors eagerly enlisted at the beginning of
the conflict but this rate declined by the midpoint of the war. As the war
progressed and more job opportunities became available at home and in
Britain, the number of Irish medical men enlisting in the British Army
medical services declined significantly and never rallied again. Numbers
of recruits dropped substantially in 1918 because by then, Ireland, akin
to Britain, could ill afford to send any more doctors into the army.

© The Author(s) 2019                                                            209
D. Durnin, *The Irish Medical Profession and the First World War*,
Medicine and Biomedical Sciences in Modern History,
https://doi.org/10.1007/978-3-030-17959-5_7

Building on the work of Fitzpatrick and Jeffery, it has been argued that Irish medical personnel were motivated to join for a variety of factors that were shared with those enlisting in the regular forces, including economic benefit and family tradition.[3] Doctors, however, had an additional set of push and pull factors that were linked more explicitly to their professional identity. They were professionally trained and had the knowledge and capabilities to treat the sizeable number of sick and wounded soldiers. The IMWC were important agents in encouraging Irish medical personnel to participate in the conflict. Horne has contended that self-mobilisation was evident throughout civilian society in Britain, France and Germany, primarily in the first two years of war.[4] It has been posited here that self-mobilisation among the members of the Irish medical profession prompted and maintained their involvement for the duration of the conflict. By establishing their own recruiting committee, doctors ensured continued involvement in the recruitment process. Indeed, medical recruitment in Ireland, as in Britain, was characterised by self-government.

It has also been reasoned that political struggles in Ireland during the First World War disrupted medical recruitment. While the Easter Rising of 1916 had the potential to interfere with rates of recruitment, it was the development of nationalist support among poor law boards of guardians in Ireland, detailed by Feingold and Crossman, and the conflict this caused with the LGBI that proved the greater threat.[5] Due to this animosity, wartime medical recruitment suffered as guardians throughout Ireland deliberately disobeyed the LGBI's rules regarding the wartime arrangements for MOs who enlisted into the army. Irish doctors thus worried for their jobs, prompting a fall in enlistment rates. Similarly, the LGBI put Irish civilian medical provision at risk by refusing to allow the guardians to appoint men of military age, even when the various unions badly required doctors. Ultimately, political struggles in Ireland complicated Irish medical involvement in the First World War.

On the battlefields, the outbreak of the Easter Rising in 1916 had the potential to harm Irish doctors' relations with their British colleagues and consequently disrupt their wartime experiences. Rees and Tyquin have argued that members of the Australian medical profession did not have wholly positive wartime experiences because British doctors and nurses discriminated against Australians due to their nationality.[6] However, it has been posited here that Irish doctors retained amiable relations with British doctors, even after the outbreak of the Easter Rising. Doctors were more concerned with the battles that surrounded them on the frontlines than events in Ireland. It is thus argued that Irish, English, Scottish and Welsh doctors shared similar wartime experiences, regardless of their nationality.

Jones' analysis of Irish medical migration from 1860 to 1905 has identified the large numbers of Irish medical graduates travelling abroad in search of employment due to the congested medical marketplace in Ireland.[7] As part of this medical migration, Irish doctors enlisted into the British Army. This study of Irish doctors' involvement in the First World War has contended that during the war, the pattern of enlistment grew considerably in an expansion of tradition. In addition, one of the notable negative effects of the wartime developments in the Irish medical profession was that the state of overcrowding reached new heights following demobilisation. From 1914 to 1918, war had acted as a release valve for the Irish medical profession. However, the effect was only for the duration of conflict and the problem of overcrowding was exacerbated following the end of war.

This study has also examined the impact of war on civilian medical provision in poor law unions and hospitals. While Winter has argued that the efficiency of recruitment procedures protected civilian medical provision, this study has suggested that such an argument, at least in the Irish case, fails to wholly consider the inner workings and state of the medical profession before the conflict. While the IMWC generally managed to balance medical recruitment well, it was largely assisted in this by the overcrowded state of the Irish medical profession prior to war. As a result, the enlistment of doctors did not wholly damage the provision of civilian health care in hospitals. In most counties in Ireland, there was a surfeit of doctors ready to occupy vacant medical roles, albeit for the temporary period of war. Foremost among them were women doctors. Kelly has argued that female doctors entered into the medical profession in Ireland thanks to the increase in opportunities due to war.[8] Extending this argument, this study posits that during the early years of the war, this influx of women doctors into jobs vacated by men enlisting into the British Army helped to reduce the impact of Irish medical involvement in the war on civilian medical infrastructure.

In addition, by the latter stages of war, when the Irish medical profession was stretched to the limit, hospital governors exploited their links with local universities and turned to medical students to alleviate staff shortages. There was, however, a noticeable shortage of doctors in Ireland in some rural poor law unions, and this was largely a result of the LGBI's employment restrictions. While young doctors continued to apply for poor law dispensary posts, they were continually rejected due to the LGBI's strict adherence to their wartime professional protectionist policies.

One of the key findings of this book is that the First World War adversely affected Irish civilian hospitals. Cooter's argument that wartime improvements to medical provision often did not extend beyond the war years has been proven true in the Irish context, at least as far as hospitals are concerned.[9] Following the signing of the Armistice, the expansion of the military and civilian hospital system in Ireland, which occurred as a consequence of war, soon reversed. Most of the hospitals and wards that had been especially established for the treatment of soldiers closed rather than continue for the benefit of civilian patients. Coleman has contended that Irish civilian hospitals, funded through voluntary subscriptions and donations, were suffering financially before the war and it has been argued here that wartime inflation further destabilised the fragile financial base of Ireland's hospital system.[10] While Irish civilian hospitals experienced significant rises in income, ultimately, the war negatively affected their financial state. In the latter years of the conflict, a decrease in philanthropic support, coupled with a rise in expenditure linked to inflation plunged the hospitals into even more financial difficulty. The evidence suggests that the rising cost of care, associated with war, and the admission of soldiers was detrimental to the civilian hospital provision.

Abel-Smith has argued that hospitals in Britain demonstrated some signs of financial recovery in the 1920s due to the support of the government and public.[11] Yet the same cannot be said about developments in Ireland. Instead, the changing political situation in Ireland ensured that the financial state of the hospitals continued to deteriorate. It was not until the 1930s, following the introduction of the Irish hospitals' sweepstake, that hospitals' finances began to improve. Therefore, Irish civilian hospitals survived the First World War but the conflict destabilised their financial health to such an extent that it fundamentally altered the provision of healthcare in hospitals in Ireland for many years after the war had ended.

## NOTES

1. Callan, 'Voluntary recruiting for the British Army in Ireland during the First World War'; Fitzpatrick, *Ireland and the First World War*, pp. 1–24.
2. Whitehead, *Doctors in the Great War*, pp. 32–90.
3. Fitzpatrick, 'The logic of collective sacrifice', pp. 1017–1030; Jeffery, *Ireland and the Great War*, pp. 5–36.
4. Horne, 'Mobilizing for Total War', p. 5.
5. Feingold, 'The tenant's movement to capture the Irish Poor Law boards, 1877–1886', p. 225; Crossman, *Politics, pauperism and power*, p. 36.
6. Rees, *The other Anzacs*, p. 211; Tyquin, *Little by little*, p. 130.
7. Jones, 'Strike out boldly', pp. 55–74.
8. Kelly, *Irish women in medicine, c.1880s–1920s*, pp. 135–158.
9. Cooter, 'Medicine and the goodness of war', pp. 147–159.
10. Coleman, *The Irish sweep*, pp. 1–15.
11. Abel-Smith, *The hospitals*, p. 323.

# APPENDICES

See Tables A1, A2, B1, B2, B3, B4, B5, C1, and C2.

**Table A1**  Full list of Central Medical War Committee members

| | |
|---|---|
| T. Jenner Verrall | BMA |
| Sir James Barr | BMA |
| H.W. Langley Browne | BMA |
| Dr. Charles Buttar | BMA |
| Dr. Adam Fulton | BMA |
| Dr. Thomas Hennessy | IMA and BMA |
| Sir Rickman J. Goldee | BMA |
| Prof. Harvey Littlejohn | BMA |
| Dr. J.A. MacDonald | BMA |
| Sir Robert Morant | National Health Insurance Commissioner |
| Dr. Edwin Rayner | BMA |
| Dr. B.A. Richmond | BMA |
| Dr. A.E. Shipley | BMA |
| Dr. S.W. Wheaton | Local Government Board |
| J. Smith Whittaker | National Health Insurance Commissioner |

*Source* CMWC minute book, 9 August 1916 (TNA, MH 47/162)

**Table A2**   Full list of Irish Medical War Committee members

| | |
|---|---|
| E. Coey Bigger | MD, Local Government Board |
| D.J. Coffey | President, University College Dublin |
| Ephraim Cosgrave | President, Royal College of Physicians of Ireland |
| Right Hon. M.F. Cox | Privy Council of Ireland |
| A.F. Dixon | Trinity College, Dublin |
| F. Conway Dwyer | President, Royal College of Surgeons of Ireland |
| Maurice Hayes | MD |
| Colonel M.L. Hearn | RAMC |
| Thomas Hennessy | British Medical Association (Ireland) |
| R.W. Leslie | Queens University Belfast |
| Lieut. J.C. McWalter | RAMC |
| W.J. Maguire | National Health Insurance Commission (Ireland) |
| H.W. Mason | Apothecaries Hall |
| A. Moore | Dean of Medical Faculty, University College Cork |
| Joseph O'Carroll | Vice President, Royal College of Physicians of Ireland |
| A.C. O'Sullivan | Trinity College, Dublin |
| J.P. Pye | University College Galway |
| Sir Thomas J. Stafford | Local Government Board |
| R.J. Rowlette | MD |
| William Taylor | Vice President RCSI |

*Source* 'Irish Medical War Committee', Central Medical War Committee minute book, MH 47 62, TNA

**Table B1**   King George V Hospital, Dublin: admissions, deaths and average daily sick (August 1914–October 1919)

| *Month* | *Admissions* | *Deaths* | *Average daily sick* |
|---|---|---|---|
| *1914* | | | |
| January | – | – | – |
| February | – | – | – |
| March | – | – | – |
| April | – | – | – |
| May | – | – | – |
| June | – | – | – |
| July | – | – | – |
| August | 152 | 3 | 128 |
| September | 345 | 2 | 203 |
| October | 455 | 5 | 231 |
| November | 427 | 2 | 249 |
| December | 448 | 3 | 249 |
| Total | 1857 | 15 | 1060 |
| Beds equipped | 244 | | |

(continued)

**Table B1** (continued)

| Month | Admissions | Deaths | Average daily sick |
|---|---|---|---|
| *1915* | | | |
| January | 367 | 4 | 439 |
| February | 579 | 4 | 439 |
| March | 567 | 4 | 368 |
| April | 476 | 2 | 380 |
| May | 303 | – | 297 |
| June | 359 | 2 | 320 |
| July | 355 | 2 | 324 |
| August | 348 | – | 299 |
| September | 360 | 1 | 315 |
| October | 340 | – | 326 |
| November | 337 | – | 317 |
| December | 350 | 4 | 306 |
| Total | 4941 | 23 | 4127 |
| Beds equipped | 512 | | |
| *1916* | | | |
| January | 472 | 1 | 351 |
| February | 440 | 5 | 403 |
| March | 530 | 5 | 379 |
| April | 390 | 3 | 333 |
| May | 861 | 2 | 378 |
| June | 645 | 3 | 481 |
| July | 563 | 1 | 485 |
| August | 471 | – | 494 |
| September | 486 | – | 529 |
| October | 604 | 1 | 606 |
| November | 536 | 2 | 626 |
| December | 542 | 2 | 606 |
| Total | 6540 | 25 | 5670 |
| Beds equipped | 851 | | |
| *1917* | | | |
| January | 422 | 4 | 628 |
| February | 318 | 4 | 632 |
| March | 325 | 5 | 630 |
| April | 294 | 5 | 591 |
| May | 345 | – | 535 |
| June | 297 | 2 | 560 |
| July | 274 | 3 | 472 |
| August | 463 | – | 512 |
| September | 397 | – | 512 |
| October | 480 | 5 | 498 |

(continued)

## Table B1   (continued)

| Month | Admissions | Deaths | Average daily sick |
|---|---|---|---|
| November | 440 | 5 | 534 |
| December | 455 | 6 | 527 |
| Total | 4500 | 39 | 6631 |
| Beds equipped | 921 | | |
| *1918* | | | |
| January | 488 | 9 | 572 |
| February | 464 | 1 | 621 |
| March | 586 | 2 | 646 |
| April | 593 | 5 | 705 |
| May | 589 | 22 | 574 |
| June | 878 | 14 | 594 |
| July | 645 | 16 | 505 |
| August | 512 | 8 | 488 |
| September | 554 | 2 | 513 |
| October | 1053 | 34 | 659 |
| November | 879 | 44 | 778 |
| December | 589 | 5 | 745 |
| Total | 7830 | 162 | 7401 |
| Beds equipped | 753 | | |
| *1919* | | | |
| January | 483 | 7 | 611 |
| February | 616 | 26 | 554 |
| March | 486 | 18 | 309 |
| April | 379 | 9 | 376 |
| May | 421 | 6 | 379 |
| June | 382 | 3 | 294 |
| July | 388 | 4 | 315 |
| August | 360 | 6 | 348 |
| September | 395 | 3 | 327 |
| October | 442 | 1 | 296 |
| November | – | – | – |
| December | – | – | – |
| Total | 4352 | 85 | 4009 |
| Beds equipped | 389 | | |

*Source* 'Report of Deputy Director of Medical Services (Irish Command)', 26 January 1920, WO 35/179, TNA

**Table B2** Military hospitals in the northern district, 1914–1918

| Military hospital | Beds in 1914 | Increased to |
|---|---|---|
| Belfast | 50 | 336 |
| Armagh | 8 | 30 |
| Dundalk | 8 | 20 |
| Enniskillen | 14 | 30 |
| Holywood | 35 | 64 |
| Londonderry | 25 | 130 |
| Omagh | 5 | 30 |
| Newry | – | 20 |
| Athlone | 10 | – |
| Mullingar | 20 | – |
| Longford | 12 | – |

*Source* 'Report of Assistant Director of Medical Services (Ulster Brigade)', 14 January 1920, WO 35/179, TNA

**Table B3** Military hospitals in the southern district, 1914–1918

| | Beds prior to war | Increased to |
|---|---|---|
| Buttevant | 16 | 41 |
| Cork | 75 | 215 |
| Fermoy | 65 | 210 |
| Limerick | 26 | 72 |
| Queenstown | 30 | 82 |
| Spike Island | 0 | 500 |
| Tipperary | 50 | 62 |
| Total | 262 | 1182 |

*Source* 'Report of Assistant Director of Medical Services (6th Division)', 16 December 1919, WO 35/179, TNA

**Table B4** Dates of convoys of sick and wounded soldiers arriving in Cork, 1914–1918

| Year | Number of convoys | Date of arrival |
|---|---|---|
| 1914 | 2 | 26 October 2014; 5 November 2014 |
| 1915 | 2 | 30 April 2015; 16 December 2015 |
| 1916 | 6 | 5 February 2016; 28 February 2016; 17 September 2016; 7 November 2016; 19 November 2016; 20 December 2016 |
| 1917 | 0 | – |
| 1918 | 3 | 21 January 2018; 11 February 2018; 26 June 2018 |

*Source* 'Report of Assistant Director of Medical Services (6th Division)', 16 December 1919, WO 35/179, TNA

**Table B5**  Auxiliary hospitals affiliated with the King George V Hospital, Dublin, during the First World War

| Hospital | Number of beds | Date of opening | Date of closing | Approximate number of cases treated during the war |
|---|---|---|---|---|
| Adelaide Civilian Hospital | 30 | 27 October 2014 | 28 February 2019 | 780 |
| Drumcondra Civilian Hospital | 10 | 15 February 2015 | 3 October 2017 | 190 |
| Dublin Castle Red Cross Hospital | 260 | 17 February 2015 | 30 April 2019 | 5160 |
| Hume Street Civilian Hospital | 30 | 16 February 2015 | 1 November 2017 | 184 |
| Irish Counties Red X Hospital, Glasnevin | 260 | 19 June 2017 | 31 May 2019 | 2149 |
| Jervis Street Civilian Hospital | 30 | 27 October 2014 | 28 February 2019 | 735 |
| Mater Hospital | 74 | 27 October 2014 | 19 February 2019 | 1118 |
| Meath Civilian Hospital, Dublin | 23 | 27 October 2014 | 28 February 2019 | 498 |
| Mercers Civilian Hospital Dublin | 28 | 27 October 2014 | 28 February 2019 | 567 |
| Mountjoy Square V.A.D. Hospital | 24 | 15 February 2015 | 1 February 2019 | 250 |
| National Children's Hospital, Dublin | 12 | 27 October 2014 | 28 February 2019 | 192 |
| Officers Hospital, Fitzwilliam Street, Dublin | 10 | 27 October 2014 | 31 March 2019 | 230 |
| Richmond Civilian Hospital | 182 | 27 October 2014 | 31 May 2019 | 2432 |
| Richmond War Hospital, Grangegorman | 32 | 27 October 2014 | – | 741 |
| Royal City of Dublin Hospital | 53 | 27 October 2014 | 23 February 2019 | 889 |
| Royal Victoria Eye and Ear Hospital | 20 | 23 October 2014 | 30 September 2019 | 349 |
| Sir Patrick Dun's Hospital | 30 | 27 October 2014 | 28 February 2019 | 432 |
| Dr. Steevens' Civilian Hospital | 71 | 27 October 2014 | | 1126 |
| St. Michael's Hospital, Kingstown | 15 | 27 October 2014 | 31 October 2017 | 271 |
| St. Vincent's Civilian Hospital | 25 | 27 October 2014 | 15 February 2019 | 425 |
| *Auxiliary convalescent hospitals* | | | | |
| Balrath Bury Auxiliary Hospital, Meath | 40 | 29 May 2017 | 11 February 2019 | 491 |
| Bloomfield Auxiliary Hospital, Mullingar | 40 | 3 May 2017 | 31 May 2019 | 501 |
| Corrig Castle Auxiliary Castle, Dublin | 42 | 1 April 2015 | 7 February 2019 | 1008 |
| Cottage Hospital, Drogheda | 10 | 5 March 2017 | 28 February 2019 | 147 |
| Duke of Connaught Hospital, Bray | 60 | 12 April 2017 | 31 July 2019 | 1680 |

(continued)

**Table B5** (continued)

| Hospital | Number of beds | Date of opening | Date of closing | Approximate number of cases treated during the war |
|---|---|---|---|---|
| Fetherstonhaugh Auxiliary Hospital, Dublin | 20 | 7 October 2016 | 17 February 2019 | 741 |
| Glenmaroon Auxiliary Hospital, Dublin | 12 | 30 October 2014 | 30 April 2019 | 430 |
| The Hermitage Hospital, Dublin | 80 | 1 April 2017 | 1 May 2019 | 674 |
| Lady Desarts Auxiliary Hospital, Kilkenny | 20 | 1 July 2017 | 31 July 2019 | 340 |
| Linden Auxiliary Hospital, Dublin | 30 | 3 November 2014 | 31 March 2019 | 950 |
| Monkstown House Auxiliary Hospital, Dublin | 50 | 1 February 2015 | 1 June 2019 | 929 |
| Officers Hospital, Tudenham Park, Mullingar | 20 | 30 August 2017 | 30 November 2018 | 180 |
| Princess Patricia Hospital, Bray | 20 | 1 May 2016 | 30 September 2019 | 2094 |
| Rockfield Auxiliary Hospital, Blackrock | 8 | 1 February 2015 | 31 March 2017 | 196 |
| Stillorgan Auxiliary Hospital, Dublin | 36 | 2 October 2016 | 6 February 2019 | 590 |
| Temple Hill Auxiliary Hospital, Blackrock | 24 | 3 February 2015 | 15 March 2019 | 694 |

*Source* 'Report of Deputy Director of Medical Services (Irish Command)', 26 January 1920, WO 35/179, TNA

**Table C1** Auxiliary Belfast area hospitals operating during the First World War

*Auxiliary military hospitals*

| Hospital | Number of beds |
|---|---|
| Waveney, Ballymena | 100 |
| UVF, Belfast | 382 |
| UVF, Gilford | 52 |
| Royal Victoria | 59 |
| Mater, Belfast | 92 |
| Ballywalter Park | 10 |
| Mount Stewart House, Newtownards | 16 |
| Railway Hospital, Whitehead | 15 |
| Whitehead King's Rd | 40 |
| Banger Cottage | 50 |
| Cushendall Cottage | 12 |
| Downpatrick County Infirmary | 20 |
| Cottage Hospital, Drogheda | 10 |
| Co.Antrim Infirmary, Lisburn | 14 |
| Newtownards Union | 100 |
| Hilden Convalescent Hospital | 122 |
| County Infirmary, Londonderry | 30 |
| VAD Hospital, Strabane | 15 |
| County Infirmary Armagh | 30 |
| Red Cross Hospital, Dundalk | 30 |
| County Infirmary, Dundalk | 20 |
| County Infirmary, Enniskillen | 30 |
| General Hospital, Newry | 9 |
| Co. Infirmary, Omagh | 30 |

*Source* 'Report of Assistant Director of Medical Services (Ulster Brigade)', 14 January 1920, WO 35/179, TNA

**Table C2** Hospital ships and their date of arrival in Dublin Port, 1914–1919

| | |
|---|---|
| H.S. Oxfordshire | 5 November 2014 |
| H.S. Carisbrooke Castle | 17 February 2015 |
| Valdivia | 19 March 2015 |
| H.S. Oxfordshire | 30 April 2015 |
| H.S. Oxfordshire | 27 June 2015 |
| H.S. Oxfordshire | 7 August 2015 |
| H.S. Oxfordshire | 4 October 2015 |
| Dover Castle | 16 December 2015 |
| Salta | 1 July 2016 |
| Marama | 22 July 2016 |
| Salta | 4 August 2016 |
| Salta | 17 August 2016 |
| Salta | 3 September 2016 |

(continued)

**Table C2**   (continued)

| | |
|---|---|
| Salta | 17 September 2016 |
| Glengorm Castle | 7 October 2016 |
| Maheno | 18 October 2016 |
| Gloucester Castle | 7 November 2016 |
| Wandinna | 20 December 2016 |
| Wandinna | 6 January 2017 |
| Barilda | 21 January 2017 |
| Essequibo | 5 February 2017 |
| Cambria | 7 June 2017 |
| Cambria | 13 June 2017 |
| Cambria | 19 June 2017 |
| Cambria | 20 June 2017 |
| Cambria | 29 June 2017 |
| Cambria | 1 July 2017 |
| Cambria | 3 July 2017 |
| Cambria | 6 July 2017 |
| Cambria | 9 July 2017 |
| Cambria | 10 July 2017 |
| Cambria | 12 July 2017 |
| Cambria | 14 August 2017 |
| Cambria | 29 September 2017 |
| Cambria | 1 October 2017 |
| Cambria | 23 October 2017 |
| Cambria | 26 November 2017 |
| Cambria | 5 December 2017 |
| Cambria | 6 December 2017 |
| Wandinna | 11 February 2018 |
| Wandinna | 11 May 2018 |
| Wandinna | 26 June 2018 |
| Brammar Castle | 23 October 2018 |
| Gurkn | 3 February 2019 |

*Source* 'Report of Deputy Director of Medical Services (Irish Command)', 26 January 1920, WO 35/179, TNA; Royal Irish Automobile Club, *War services presented to S.P. Anderson as a record of assistance given in connection with the wounded soldier's reception committee* (Dublin 1919)

# SELECT BIBLIOGRAPHY

## PRIMARY SOURCES

**Manuscript**
*British Red Cross Archive, London*
Personnel Indexes, 1914–1918.

*Department of Manuscripts, the National Library of Ireland, Dublin*
Diary of Mrs. Augustine Henry (Alice Helen Brunton) for the period August 1914 to July 1919, vols. 1–8, Ms. 7981–Ms. 7988.
Diaries of Major S.M. Adye-Curran of the Royal Army Medical Corps, 1914–1919, vols. 1–3, Ms. 34393.
Postcards to his family in Ireland from Doran of Dublin serving with the Royal Army Medical Corps in France, *c.* 1916–1918, Ms. 24581.

*Imperial War Museum, London*
Pocket diary of Bruce West, PP/MCR/335.
Audio recordings of interviews with Irish nurse who participated in the First World War: IWM/739; IWM/917; IWM/5395; IWM/6845.

*Irish Military Archives, Dublin*
Bureau of Military History records:
Witness statement of Sean MacEoin, WS1716.

© The Editor(s) (if applicable) and The Author(s),
under exclusive license to Springer Nature Switzerland AG 2019
D. Durnin, *The Irish Medical Profession and the First World War*,
Medicine and Biomedical Sciences in Modern History,
https://doi.org/10.1007/978-3-030-17959-5

Witness statement of Sean Fitzgibbon, WS30.
Witness statement of Michael O'Dea, WS1152.

*Manuscripts and Archives Research Library, Trinity College, Dublin*
The papers of James Johnston Abraham, 1876–1963, MS 11007.
Papers of Major Richard William George Hingston, 1912–1928, MSS 10484/1-9.

*National Archives of Ireland*
Meath Hospital minute book, 1913–1925, 2007/128.
Monkstown Hospital minute book, 1913–1925, 2006/96.
Royal City of Dublin Hospital minute book, 1913–1925, 2006/98.
North Dublin Union Workhouse minute book, 1912–1918, MFGS 49/128.
South Dublin Union Workhouse minute book, 1912–1920, MFGS 49/89.
Rathdown Union Workhouse minute book, 1912–1918, MFGS 49/91.
Richmond District Asylum book of newspaper cuttings, uncatalogued.
Richmond War Hospital minute book, 1915–1919, uncatalogued.

*National Archives, UK*
Service records of women who served in Queen Alexandra's Imperial Military
    Nursing Service and Territorial Force Nursing Service during the First World
    War, 1914–1918, WO399.
Central Medical War Committee minutes, 1914–1918, MH 47/162.
Report of Deputy Director of Medical Services, Irish Command, 26 January
    1920, WO 35 179.

*Parliamentary Debates*
Dáil Éireann debates.

*Public Records Office of Northern Ireland, Belfast, Co. Antrim*
First World War nursing diaries of Miss Emma Duffin, vols. 1–5, 1915–1917,
    D2109/18/4.
Correspondence of Miss Emma Duffin, 1915–1917, D2109/9; D2109/10/1D;
    D2109/11; D2109/18.
Lady Hermione Blackwood's letters to her mother recounting her experiences as
    a nurse in France in the First World War, 1915, D1231/G/7.
Correspondence concerning a hospital ward and recreation room at a Red
    Cross Hospital in Nottingham support by the Orange Order in Ireland,
    1916–1918, D2023/11/1A.
Intimidation of Catholic ex-servicemen in Craigavon Hospital, 1922, CAB/6/9.
Volume containing details of soldiers treated at the Royal Victoria Hospital,
    1914–1916, HOS/2/1/4/1.
Alleged attack by Crown Forces on the Mater Hospital, 1922, CAB/6/47.
Medical Staff minute book for Royal Victoria Hospital, 1912–1925,
    HOS/2/1/1/2/3.
Hospital care for ex-servicemen, 36th (Ulster) Division, 1923–1937,
    CAB/9/G/65.

Letters to and from Matthew McCaul, Chaplain with 1st Highland Light Infantry in Mesopotamia, and Lt George Barton McCaul MC, Royal Army Medical Corps on the Salonika Front, 1918, D1893.

Reminiscences of Robert Whelan (written in 1963) including an account of the Easter rising in Dublin when Whelan served as a Red Cross volunteer, 1916, D3041.

Correspondence concerning a hospital ward and recreation room at a Red Cross Hospital in Nottingham support by the Orange Order in Ireland, 1916–1918, D2023/11/1A.

Ulster Volunteer Force Hospital, Belfast, D1898/1/58A.

Management Committee minute book for Royal Victoria Hospital 1906–1916, MIC514/1/1/20.

Management Committee minute book for Royal Victoria Hospital 1916–1924, MIC514/1/1/21.

Medical Staff minute book for Royal Victoria Hospital, MIC514/1/2/3.

*Royal College of Physicians of Ireland Heritage Centre*
Book of Sir Patrick Dun's Hospital, 1909–1923, PDH/1/2/1/9-10.

Dublin Castle Hospital minute book, 1914–1919, BMS/5.

Dublin Clinical Hospitals Committee correspondence, 1914, DCHC/2/14.

Publicity flyer for the Irish Counties War Hospital, 1917, TPCK/6/6/10.

The Kirkpatrick Index, TPCK/5/3.

*Royal College of Surgeons in Ireland Heritage Centre*
Book of newspaper cuttings, uncatalogued.

Minutes of the council, 1912–1919, uncatalogued.

Hospital for wounded officers, minute book, 1914–1918.

*Wellcome Library, London*
The Royal Army Medical Corps Muniment collection:

Portrait photo of David Ahern, RAMC 1946.

Portrait photo of Ralph Ainsworth, RAMC 1168.

Health memoranda for soldiers by Lieutenant Colonel H.K. Allport, RAMC 230; RAMC 729/3; RAMC 1638/2.

History of 217 Field Ambulance, diary/scrapbook of Lieutenant Colonel R.A. Anderson, RAMC, the unit's first commanding officer, RAMC 732.

Portrait photo of William Ormsby Ball, RAMC 801/22/18.

Papers of General R.J. Blackham, RAMC, bound into one volume, RAMC 588; RAMC 589.

Typescript copy of the diary of Captain Brett, RAMC, on H.M. Hospital Ship Oxfordshire in the Dardanelles, November 1915–January 1916, written as a letter to "Katie", RAMC 1595.

Message from the officer commanding 6th Division, re distinguished conduct of Private Edward George Brown, RAMC 1827.

Portrait photo of Charles Buckly, RAMC 2091.

Commission of Maurice Burnett as Lieutenant in the RAMC. With certificate of mention in despatches, 1915, and an extract from the "Radio Times", 1929, re the Battle of Shaiba, Mesopotamia, in which Burnett was killed, RAMC 1018.
Papers of surgeon general William Francis Burnett, RAMC 1263; RAMC 2091.
Papers of Charles Henry Burtchaell, RAMC 364/2; RAMC 446; RAMC 591; RAMC 1165/2.
Papers of Lieutenant Colonel Herbert St. Maur Carter, RAMC 793.
Papers and photographs of Brigadier William Pennefather Croker, RAMC, RAMC 1907.
Papers of Colonel Sir William Donovan, RAMC 523.
Biographical notes re major general John Dallas Edge, RAMC, with correspond-ence, 1929–1930, including Edge's own account of his leadership in the defence of Orange Walk, Honduras, RAMC 52/4.
Bound volume of 11 articles and pamphlets written by George Evatt, RAMC 181; RAMC 423; RAMC 474; RAMC 523/13; RAMC 653.
Portrait photo of William Foot, RAMC 1328.
Interview with James Stewart Gallie, RAMC 1165/2/4.
Letter from Thomas Gibbon to his brother, RAMC 535.
Portrait photo of Sir James Hartigan, RAMC 2011.
Papers of Sir Anthony Bowlby, consulting surgeon to the British Armies in France during the First World War, RAMC 365; RAMC 448; RAMC 761/2/10; RAMC 801/6/4; RAMC 1799.
Captain J.P. Lynch's accounts of his experiences in the First World War, RAMC 453.
The works of Sir W. MacArthur, RAMC 644; RAMC 812; RAMC 2091.
Certificates of captain John Smith McCombe, RAMC, RAMC 389.
Certificate of mention in despatches of Robert McKinlay, RAMC 538.
Certificates and diplomas of Lieutenant Colonel Campbell McQueen, RAMC 1084.
Souvenirs of major general Jeremiah John Magner, RAMC, RAMC 1764.
Papers of Lieutenant general Sir Thomas O'Donnell, RAMC 859.
Draft letter by Sir Henry Rawlinson, RAMC 739/16.
Five certificates of mention of Colonel (later major-general) H.N. Thompson, RAMC, in despatches, 1915–1919, RAMC 1955.

CONTEMPORARY PUBLISHED SOURCES

*The Belvederian*, 1912–1925.
*Ireland's memorial records, 1914–18: Being the names of Irishmen who fell in the Great European War.* Dublin, 1923.
*Medical Directories for Ireland*, 1852–1925.
*War list and roll of honour of the National University of Ireland.* Dublin, 1919.
Abraham, James Johnston. *Surgeon's journey.* London, 1957.

Black, Catherine. *King's nurse, beggar's nurse*. London, 1939.

Dawson, W.R. 'The work of the Belfast War Hospital' in *British Journal of Psychiatry*, 71 (1925), pp. 219–24.

MacKinnon, Albert. *Malta: The nurse of the Mediterranean*. London, 1916.

MacPherson, William. *History of the Great War based on official documents: Medical services*. London, 1921.

Order of St. John of Jerusalem. *The Red Cross in Ireland: An account of the Red Cross work of the St. John Ambulance Brigade and the British Red Cross Society in Leinster, Munster and Connaught: From 1 Aug. 1914 to Nov. 1918*. Dublin, 1920.

Royal Irish Automobile Club. *War services presented to S.P. Anderson as a record of assistance given in connection with the wounded soldier's reception committee*. Dublin, 1919.

*British Medical Journal*, 1858–1936:

Anon. 'The week' in *British Medical Journals*, 4-1, no. 95 (1858), p. 889.

Anon. 'Army Medical Department' in *British Medical Journal*, 904, no. 1 (1878), p. 615.

Anon. 'Summary of the Royal Commission on South African Hospitals' in *British Medical Journal*, 2091, no. 1 (1901), p. 236.

Anon. 'Ireland' in *British Medical Journal*, 2798, no. 2 (1914), p. 346.

Anon. 'Tribute to the work of the RAMC' in *British Medical Journal*, 2814, no. 2 (1914), p. 984.

Anon. 'Trinity College, Dublin and the war' in *British Medical Journal*, 2814, no. 2 (1914), p. 996.

Anon. 'Medical War Committee' in *British Medical Journal*, 2823, no. 1 (1915), p. 268.

Anon. 'Medical students and the war' in *British Medical Journal*, 2861, no. 2 (1915), p. 648.

Anon. 'Central Medical War Committee' in *British Medical Journal*, 2865, no. 2 (1915), p. 785.

Anon. 'Poor Law Medical Officers on military service' in *British Medical Journal*, 2860, no. 2 (1915), p. 622.

Anon. 'Lord French's dispatch' in *British Medical Journal*, 2872, no. 1 (1916), p. 109.

Anon. 'Conditions of leave to Poor Law Medical Officers joining the Royal Army Medical Corps' in *British Medical Journal*, 2874, no. 1 (1916), p. 181.

Anon. 'Medical recruiting' in *British Medical Journal*, 2875, no. 1 (1916), p. 214.

Anon. 'Irish Medical War Committee' in *British Medical Journal*, 2877, no. 1 (1916), p. 289.

Anon. 'Recruiting' in *British Medical Journal*, 2877, no. 1 (1916), p. 287.

Anon. 'Recruiting for the Naval and Military Medical Services' in *British Medical Journal*, 2877, no. 1 (1916), p. 617.

Anon. 'The report of the Royal Commission on venereal diseases' in *British Medical Journal*, 2880, no. 1 (1916), p. 380.

Anon. 'Irish Medical War Committee' in *British Medical Journal*, 2879, no. 1 (1916), p. 359.

Anon. 'Ireland' in *British Medical Journal*, 2890, no. 1 (1916), p. 738.

Anon. 'Base Hospitals in Egypt' in *British Medical Journal*, 2916, no. 2 (1916), p. 702.

Anon. 'Ireland' in *British Medical Journal*, 2916, no. 2 (1916), p. 702.

Anon. 'Dublin Hospital Sunday' in *British Medical Journal*, 2939, no. 1 (1917), p. 563.

Anon. 'Dublin Hospital staff for France' in *British Medical Journal*, 2941, no. 1 (1917), p. 631.

Anon. 'Hospital ships for the Tigris' in *British Medical Journal*, 2946, no. 1 (1917), p. 819.

Anon. 'Craigavon Neurasthenic Hospital for soldiers, Belfast' in *British Medical Journal*, 2952, no. 2 (1917), p. 132.

Anon. 'Deputy surgeon-general William Cherry, RAMC' in *British Medical Journal*, 2964, no. 2 (1917), p. 541.

Anon. 'Ireland' in *British Medical Journal*, 2966, no. 2 (1917), p. 602.

Anon. 'Ireland' in *British Medical Journal*, 2968, no. 2 (1917), p. 668.

Anon. 'Ireland' in *British Medical Journal*, 3011, no. 2 (1918), p. 299.

Anon. 'Immediate need of doctors for the army' in *British Medical Journal*, 3015, no. 2 (1918), p. 417.

Anon. 'Medical demobilisation' in *Supplement to the British Medical Journal*, 3028, no. 1 (1919), p. 53.

Anon. 'The Central Medical War Committee and medical demobilization' in *British Medical Journal*, 3031, no. 1 (1919), p. 134.

Anon. 'Royal Victoria Hospital, Belfast' in *British Medical Journal*, 3033, no. 1 (1919), p. 199.

Anon. 'The Irish Medical War Committee' in *British Medical Journal*, 3044, no. 1 (1919), p. 560.

Anon. 'Shortage of doctors' in *British Medical Journal*, 3054, no. 2 (1919), p. 64.

Anon. 'Dublin Hospitals' in *British Medical Journal*, 3059, no. 2 (1919), p. 218.

Anon. 'Irish Public Health Council' in *British Medical Journal*, 3118, no. 2 (1920), p. 527.

Anon. 'Reports on wounded in Dublin Hospitals' in *British Medical Journal*, 3139, no. 1 (1921), p. 319.

Anon. 'Ireland' in *British Medical Journal*, 3142, no. 1 (1921), p. 439.

Anon. 'Wounded in hospital' in *British Medical Journal*, 3143, no. 1 (1921), p. 477.

Anon. 'Loss to Irish Hospitals' in *British Medical Journal*, 3176, no. 2 (1921), p. 813.

Anon. 'Appointment of Medical Officer' in *British Medical Journal*, 3217, no. 2 (1922), p. 400.

Anon. 'Meath Hospital, Dublin' in *British Medical Journal*, 3258, no. 1 (1923), p. 993.

Anon. 'Free State Army medical service' in *British Medical Journal*, 3249, no. 1 (1923), p. 609.

Anon. 'Meath Hospital, Dublin' in *British Medical Journal*, 3258, no. 1 (1923), p. 993.

Anon. 'Hospital grants and public health legislation' in *British Medical Journal*, 3258, no. 1 (1923), p. 993.

Anon. 'Sir Patrick Dun's Hospital' in *British Medical Journal*, 3322, no. 2 (1924), p. 388.

Anon. 'Sir William Launcelotte Gubbins' in *British Medical Journal*, 3371, no. 2 (1925), p. 274.

Anon. 'Dr Harold Saunderson sugars' in *British Medical Journal*, 3567, no. 1 (1929), p. 935.

Anon. 'Obituary: Lieut.-Colonel John Patrick Joseph Murphy, RAMC' in *British Medical Journal*, 3716, no. 1 (1932), p. 596.

Anon. 'Sir Thomas Gallwey' in *British Medical Journal*, 3765, no. 1 (1933), p. 393.

Anon. 'Sir Joseph Chambers' in *British Medical Journal*, 3900, no. 2 (1935), p. 648.

Anon. 'Sir F. Conway Dwyer, M.D., F.R.C.S.I' in *British Medical Journal*, 3902, no. 2 (1935), p. 765.

Anon. 'Thomas Hennessy' in *British Medical Journal*, 3914, no. 1 (1936), p. 87.

Anon. 'Sir Alfred Keogh' in *British Medical Journal*, 3944, no. 2 (1936), p. 317.

Barrett, James. 'Trachoma and visual standards during the war' in *British Medical Journal*, 2953, no. 2 (1917), p. 97.

Captain, T.F. 'The future of the medical profession' in *British Medical Journal*, 2925, no. 1 (1917), p. 86.

Hennessy, Thomas. 'Irish Medical War Committee' in *British Medical Journal*, 2864, no. 2 (1915), p. 764.

*Dublin Journal of Medical Science*, 1914–1920

Anon. 'Professional classes war relief council' in *Dublin Journal of Medical Science*, 516, no. 138 (1914).

Barlas, A.R. 'War time economy: A medical grievance' in *Dublin Journal of Medical Science*, 539, no. 142 (1916).

Benson, C. 'The effect of the war on the medical profession' in *Dublin Journal of Medical Science*, 530, no. 141 (1916).

Brereton, F.S. 'The Great War and the RAMC' in *Dublin Journal of Medical Science*, no. 3 (1920).

Burtchaell, Sir Charles. 'Disease as affecting success in the war' in *Dublin Journal of Medical Science*, 571, no. 148 (1919).

Dwyer, F.C. 'The Royal College of Surgeons in Ireland and the war' in *Dublin Journal of Medical Science*, 527, no. 140 (1915).

Gordon, Thomas E. 'The Great European War', in *Dublin Journal of Medical Science*, 517, no. 139 (1915).

## NEWSPAPERS

*Anglo-Celt*, 1912–1925.
*Belfast Evening Telegraph*, 1912–1925.
*Belfast Weekly News*, 1912–1925.
*Belfast Weekly Telegraph*, 1912–1925.
*Connacht Tribune*, 1912–1925.
*Dublin Evening Mail*, 1912–1925.
*Enniscorthy Guardian*, 1912–1925.
*Freeman's Journal*, 1912–1925.
*The Irish Independent*, 1912–1925.
*The Irish Times*, 1912–1925.
*Leitrim Observer*, 1912–1925.
*Meath Chronicle*, 1912–1925.
*Munster Express*, 1912–1925.
*Nenagh Guardian*, 1912–1925.
*Southern Star*, 1913–1925.
*The Sunday Independent*, 1912–1925.
*Tuam Herald*, 1912–1925.
*Westmeath Examiner*, 1912–1925.

## OFFICIAL PUBLICATIONS

Census of Ireland, 1901 (www.census.nationalarchives.ie) (accessed in November 2011).

Census of Ireland, 1911 (www.census.nationalarchives.ie) (accessed in November 2011).

## OFFICIAL REPORTS

*Annual reports of the Board of Superintendence of the Dublin Hospitals*, 1912–1922.
*Annual reports of the Local Government Board for Ireland*, 1912–1922.
*Annual reports of the Richmond District Lunatic Asylum medical superintendent*, 1914–1920.

*Monkstown Hospital annual reports*, 1913–1925.
*Report of the Irish Public Health Council on the public health services in Ireland*, 1919.
*Royal City of Dublin Hospital annual reports*, 1913–1925.
*Royal College of Surgeons in Ireland annual reports*, 1913–1925.
*Sir Patrick Dun's Hospital annual reports*, 1912–1925.
*The general annual reports on the British Army*, 1914–1922.

SECONDARY SOURCES

Journal Articles and Book Chapters
Barger, A.C., Benison, S., and Wolfe, E.L. 'Walter B. Cannon and the mystery of shock: A study of Anglo-American co-operation in World War 1'. *Medical History* 35 (1991), pp. 217–49.
Beardsley, Edward. 'Allied against sin: American and British responses to venereal disease in World War 1'. *Medical History* 20 (1976), pp. 189–202.
Bew, Paul. 'The politics of war'. In *Our war: Ireland and the Great War*, edited by John Horne, pp. 95–130. Dublin: Royal Irish Academy, 2008.
Bogzac, Ted. 'War neuroses and social-cultural change in England, 1914–22: The work of the War Office Committee into Shell shock'. *Journal of Contemporary History* 24 (1989), pp. 227–56.
Bourke, Joanna. 'Irish tommies: The construction of a martial manhood, 1914–18'. *Bullan* 6 (1997), pp. 13–30.
Bourke, Joanna. 'Wartime'. In *Companion to medicine in the twentieth century*, edited by Roger Cooter and John Pickstone, pp. 589–600. London: Routledge, 2000.
Bourke, Joanna. 'Shell-shock, psychiatry and the Irish soldier during the First World War'. In *Ireland and the Great War: A war to unite us all?* edited by Adrien Gregory and Senia Paseta, pp. 155–71. Manchester: Manchester University Press, 2002.
Bowman, Timothy. 'The Irish recruiting campaign and anti-recruiting campaigns 1914–18'. In *Propaganda, political rhetoric and identity, 1300–2000*, edited by Bertrand Taithe and Tim Thornton, pp. 223–38. Stroud: Sutton Publishing, 1999.
Broadberry, Stephen, and Howlett, Peter. 'The United Kingdom during World War I: Business as usual?' In *The economics of World War One*, edited by Stephen Broadberry and Mark Harrison, pp. 206–34. Cambridge: Cambridge University Press, 2005.
Brockliss, Laurence. 'Medicine, religion and social mobility in eighteenth and early nineteenth century Ireland'. In *Ireland and medicine in the seventeenth and eighteenth centuries*, edited by James Kelly and Fiona Clark, pp. 73–109. Surrey: Ashgate, 2010.

Brown, Spencer. 'British Army surgeons commissioned 1840–1909 with West Indian/West African service: A prosopographical evaluation'. *Medical History* 37 (1993), pp. 411–31.

Bull, Phillip. 'Sacrifice, liberalism and the Great War: The case of Ireland'. *War and Society* 23 (2005), pp. 13–21.

Burke, Tom. 'Rediscovery and reconciliation: The Royal Dublin Fusiliers Association'. In *Towards commemoration: Ireland in war and revolution 1912–23*, edited by John Horne and Edward Madigan, pp. 98–104. Dublin: Royal Irish Academy, 2013.

Byrne, Fiachra. '"The report of a nightmare": Hallucinating conflict in the political and personal frontiers of Ulster during the IRA border campaign of 1920–22'. In *Medicine, health and Irish experiences of conflict, 1914–45*, edited by David Durnin and Ian Miller, pp. 109–24. Manchester: Manchester University Press, 2017.

Callan, Patrick. 'British recruitment in Ireland, 1914–18'. *Revue Internationale d'Histoire Militaire* 63 (1985), pp. 41–50.

Callan, Patrick. 'Ambivalence towards the Saxon Shilling: The attitudes of the Catholic Church in Ireland towards enlistment during the First World War'. *Archivum Hibernicum* 41 (1986), pp. 99–111.

Callan, Patrick. 'Recruiting for the British Army in Ireland during the First World War'. *The Irish Sword* 17 (1987), pp. 42–56.

Charters, Erica. 'Military medicine and the ethics of war'. *Canadian Bulletin for the History of Medicine* 27 (2010), pp. 273–98.

Clark, Paul. 'Two traditions and the places between'. In *Towards commemoration: Ireland in war and revolution 1912–23*, edited by John Horne and Edward Madigan, pp. 67–73. Dublin: Royal Irish Academy, 2013.

Clear, Caitriona. 'Fewer ladies, more women'. In *Our war: Ireland and the Great War*, edited by John Horne, pp. 157–81. Dublin: Royal Irish Academy, 2008.

Codd, Pauline. 'Recruiting and responses to the war in Wexford'. In *Ireland and the First World War*, edited by David Fitzpatrick, pp. 15–26. Dublin: Lilliput Press, 1998.

Cooter, Roger. 'Medicine and the goodness of war'. *Canadian Bulletin of Medical History* 12 (1990), pp. 147–59.

Cooter, Roger. 'War and modern medicine'. In *Companion encyclopaedia of the history of medicine*, edited by William Bynum and Roy Porter, pp. 1536–73. London: Routledge, 1994.

Cooter, Roger. 'Medicine in war'. In *Medicine transformed: Health, disease and society in Europe, 1800–1930*, edited by Deborah Brunton, pp. 331–63. Manchester: Manchester University Press, 2004.

Cox, Catherine. 'Access and authority: The medical dispensary service in post-famine Ireland'. In *Cultures of care in Irish medical history, 1750–1970*, edited by Catherine Cox and Maria Luddy, pp. 57–78. London: Palgrave Macmillan, 2010.

Cox, Catherine. 'Health and welfare in Enniscorthy, 1850–1920'. In *Enniscorthy: A history*, edited by Colm Toibin, pp. 228–56. Wexford: Wexford County Council Public Service Library, 2010.

Cox, Catherine. 'The medical marketplace and medical tradition in nineteenth century Ireland'. In *Folk healing and health care practices in Britain and Ireland: Stethoscopes, wands and crystals*, edited by Ronnie Moore and Stuart McClean, pp. 55–79. Oxford: Berghahn Books, 2010.

Cox, Catherine. 'A better known territory? Medical history and Ireland'. *Proceedings of the Royal Irish Academy, Section C* 113 (2013), pp. 341–62.

Crean, Thomas. 'Labour and politics in Kerry during the First World War'. *Saothar* 19 (1994), pp. 27–39.

Cullen, Clara. 'War work on the Home Front: The Central Sphagnum Depot for Ireland at the Royal College of Science for Ireland, 1915–19'. In *Medicine, health and Irish experiences of conflict, 1914–45*, edited by David Durnin and Ian Miller, pp. 155–70. Manchester: Manchester University Press, 2017.

Daly, Mary E. 'An atmosphere of sturdy independence: The state and the Dublin Hospitals in the 1930s'. In *Medicine, disease and the state in Ireland*, edited by Elizabeth Malcolm and Greta Jones, pp. 234–52. Cork: Cork University Press, 1999.

Daly, Mary E. 'Local appointments'. In *County and town: One hundred years of local government in Ireland*, edited by Mary E. Daly, pp. 45–55. Dublin: Institute of Public Administration, 2001.

Dooney, Laura. 'Trinity College and the war'. In *Ireland and the First World War*, edited by David Fitzpatrick, pp. 36–49. Dublin: Lilliput Press, 1998.

Downes, Margaret. 'The civilian voluntary aid effort'. In *Ireland and the First World War*, edited by David Fitzpatrick, pp. 27–37. Dublin: Lilliput Press, 1998.

Doyle, Barry. 'Labour and hospitals in three Yorkshire towns: Middlesbrough, Leeds, Sheffield, 1919–1938'. *Social History of Medicine* 23 (2010), pp. 374–92.

Doyle, Barry. 'The economics, culture and politics of hospital contributory schemes: The case of inter war Leeds'. *Labour History Review* 77 (2012), pp. 289–315.

Durnin, David. '"Medicine in the city": The impact of the National Insurance Act on health care and the medical profession in Dublin'. In *A capital in conflict: Dublin City and the 1913 Lockout*, edited by Mary Clark, Francis Devine, and Máire Kennedy, pp. 83–106. Dublin: Dublin City Council, 2013.

Durnin, David. 'Ireland's British Army doctors and the treatment of Irish nationalists, 1916–23'. In *Medicine, health and Irish experiences of conflict, 1914–45*, edited by David Durnin and Ian Miller, pp. 94–108. Manchester: Manchester University Press, 2017.

Earner-Byrne, Lindsey. 'The boat to England: An analysis of the official reactions to the emigration of single Irishwomen to Britain, 1922–72'. *Irish Economic and Social History* 30 (2003), pp. 52–70.

Feingold, William L. 'The tenant's movement to capture the Irish Poor Law Boards, 1877–1886'. *Albion: A Quarterly Journal Concerned with British Studies* 7 (1975), pp. 216–31.

Fell, Alison S., and Hallett, Christine E. 'Introduction'. In *First World War nursing: New perspectives*, edited by Alison S. Fell and Christine E. Hallett, pp. 1–16. London: Taylor & Francis, 2013.

Fitzpatrick, David. 'The logic of collective sacrifice: Ireland and the British Army, 1914–18'. *Historical Journal* 38 (1995), pp. 1017–30.

Fitzpatrick, David. 'Militarism in Ireland, 1900–22'. In *A military history of Ireland*, edited by Thomas Bartlett and Keith Jeffery, pp. 379–406. Cambridge: Cambridge University Press, 1996.

Foley, Ronan. 'From front to home and back again: Geographical networks of auxiliary medical care in the First World War'. In *Medicine, health and Irish experiences of conflict, 1914–45*, edited by David Durnin and Ian Miller, pp. 125–38. Manchester: Manchester University Press, 2017.

Froggatt, Peter. 'The distinctiveness of Belfast medicine and its medical school'. *Ulster Medical Journal* 54 (1985), pp. 89–108.

Garvin, Tom. 'The Dáil Government and Irish local democracy, 1919–23'. In *County and town: One hundred years of local government in Ireland*, edited by Mary E. Daly, pp. 24–34. Dublin: Institute of Public Administration, 2001.

Gerwarth, Robert. 'The continuum of violence'. In *The Cambridge history of the First World War: The state*, edited by Jay Winter, pp. 638–62. Cambridge: Cambridge University Press, 2014.

Graffin, Seán. 'Hope and experience: Nurses from Belfast Hospitals in the First World War'. In *Medicine, health and Irish experiences of conflict, 1914–45*, edited by David Durnin and Ian Miller, pp. 125–38. Manchester: Manchester University Press, 2017.

Graubard, Stephen Richards. 'Military demobilization in Great Britain following the First World War'. *The Journal of Modern History* 19 (1947), pp. 297–311.

Halifax, Stuart. '"Over by Christmas": British popular opinion and the short war in 1914'. *First World War Studies* 1 (2010), pp. 103–21.

Hall, Lesly A. '"War always brings it on": War, STDs, the military, and the civilian population in Britain, 1850–1950'. In *Medicine and modern warfare*, edited by Roger Cooter, Mark Harrison, and Steve Sturdy, pp. 205–24. Atlanta: Clio Medica, 1999.

Harrison, Mark. 'The British Army and the problem of venereal disease in France and Egypt during the First World War'. *Medical History* 39 (1995), pp. 133–58.

Harrison, Mark. 'The fight against disease in the Mesopotamia campaign'. In *Facing Armageddon: The First World War experienced*, edited by Hugh Cecil and Peter Liddle, pp. 475–89. Barnsley: Pen and Sword Military, 1996.

Harrison, Mark. 'Medicine and the management of modern warfare'. *History of Science* 34 (1996), pp. 379–410.

Harrison, Mark. 'The medicalization of war—The militarization of medicine'. *Social History of Medicine* 9 (1996), pp. 267–76.

Harrison, Mark. 'Disease, discipline and dissent: The Indian Army in France and England, 1914–1915'. In *Medicine and modern warfare*, edited by Roger Cooter, Mark Harrison, and Steve Sturdy, pp. 185–204. Amsterdam: Clio Medica, 1999.

Horgan-Ryan, Siobhan. 'Irish military nursing in the Great War'. In *Care to remember: Nursing and midwifery in Ireland*, edited by Gerard M. Fealy, pp. 79–102. Cork: Mercier Press, 2005.

Horne, John. 'Mobilizing for total war, 1914–1918'. In *State, society and mobilization in Europe during the First World War*, edited by John Horne, pp. 1–18. Cambridge: Cambridge University Press, 1997.

Horne, John. 'Remobilizing for total war: France and Britain, 1917–1918'. In *State, society and mobilization in Europe during the First World War*, edited by John Horne, pp. 195–211. Cambridge: Cambridge University Press, 1997.

Horne, John. 'James Connolly and the great divide: Ireland, Europe and the First World War'. *Saothar* 31 (2006), pp. 75–84.

Hughes, Jonathan. '"The matchbox on a muffin": The design of hospitals in the early NHS'. *Medical History* 44 (2000), pp. 21–56.

Jones, Greta. '"Strike out boldly for the prizes that are available to you": Medical emigration from Ireland, 1860–1905'. *Medical History* 54 (2010), pp. 55–74.

Jones, Heather. 'Church of Ireland Great War remembrance in the South of Ireland: A personal reflection'. In *Towards commemoration: Ireland in war and revolution 1912–23*, edited by John Horne and Edward Madigan, pp. 74–82. Dublin: Royal Irish Academy, 2013.

Kelly, Laura. 'Migration and medical education: Irish medical students at the University of Glasgow, 1859–1900'. *Irish Economic and Social History* 31 (2012), pp. 41–62.

Kennerk, Barry. 'In danger and distress: Presentation of gunshot cases to Dublin Hospitals during the height of Fenianism, 1866–71'. *Social History of Medicine* 24 (2011), pp. 588–607.

Koven, Seth. 'Remembering and dismemberment: Crippled children, wounded soldiers and the Great War in Great Britain'. *American Historical Review* 44 (1994), pp. 1167–202.

Lawrence, Christopher. 'Continuity in crisis: Medicine, 1914–45'. In *The western medical tradition, 1800 to 2000*, edited by W.F. Bynum, Anne Hardy, Stephen

Jacyna, Christopher Lawrence, and E.M. Tansey, pp. 247–404. Cambridge: Cambridge University Press, 2006.

Leonard, Jane. 'Getting them at last: The I.R.A. and ex-servicemen'. In *Revolution? Ireland 1917–23*, edited by David Fitzpatrick, pp. 118–29. Dublin: Trinity History Workshop Publications, 1990.

Leonard, Jane. 'Facing the finger of scorn: Veteran's memories of Ireland in the twentieth century'. In *War and memory in the twentieth century*, edited by Martin Edwards and Kenneth Lunn, pp. 59–72. Oxford: Berg, 1997.

Leonard, Jane. 'Lest we forget'. In *Ireland and the First World War*, edited by David Fitzpatrick, pp. 59–67. Dublin: Lilliput Press, 1998.

Leonard, Jane. 'The Catholic Chaplaincy'. In *Ireland and the First World War*, edited by David Fitzpatrick, pp. 1–16. Dublin: Lilliput Press, 1998.

Leonard, Jane. 'Survivors'. In *Our war: Ireland and the Great War*, edited by John Horne, pp. 211–31. Dublin: Royal Irish Academy, 2008.

Lerner, Paul. 'Psychiatry and casualties of war in Germany, 1914–18'. *Journal of Contemporary History* 35 (2000), pp. 13–28.

Loudon, Irvine. 'Two thousand medical men in 1847'. *Bulletin of the Society for the Social History of Medicine* 33 (1983), pp. 4–8.

Lucey, Donnacha Seán, and Gosling, George Campbell. 'Paying for health: Comparative perspectives on patient payment and contributions for hospital provision in Ireland'. In *Healthcare in Ireland and Britain from 1850*, edited by Donnacha Seán Lucey and Virginia Crossman, pp. 81–101. London: Institute of Historical Research, 2014.

Lucey, Seán. '"These schemes will win for themselves the confidence of the people": Irish independence, poor law reform and hospital provision'. *Medical History* 58 (2014), pp. 46–66.

Luddy, Maria. 'Sex and the single girl in 1920s and 1930s Ireland'. *The Irish Review* 35 (2007), pp. 79–91.

Malcolm, Elizabeth, and Jones, Greta. 'Introduction'. In *Medicine, disease and the state in Ireland, 1650–1940*, edited by Elizabeth Malcolm and Greta Jones, pp. 1–20. Cork: Cork University Press, 1999.

Malcolm, Elizabeth. 'The Irish policeman abroad'. In *Ireland abroad: Politics and professions in the nineteenth century*, edited by Oonagh Walsh, pp. 95–107. Dublin: Four Courts Press, 2003.

Martin, F.X. '1916—Myth, fact and mystery'. *Studia Hibernica* 7 (1967), pp. 7–125.

McCormick, Leanne. 'The dangers and temptations of the street: Managing female behaviour in Belfast during the First World War'. *Women's History Review* 27 (2018), pp. 414–31.

Marsh, Patricia. 'The war and influenza: The impact of the First World War on the 1918–19 influenza pandemic in Ulster'. In *Medicine, health and Irish experiences of conflict, 1914–45*, edited by David Durnin and Ian Miller, pp. 31–44. Manchester: Manchester University Press, 2017.

Martin, Peter. 'Why have a Catholic Hospital at all? The Mater Infirmorum Hospital Belfast and the state, 1883–1972'. In *Healthcare in Ireland and Britain from 1850*, edited by Donnacha Seán Lucey and Virginia Crossman, pp. 101–16. London: Institute of Historical Research, 2014.

Matthews, Ann. 'Cumann na mBan and the Red Cross, 1914–16'. In *Associational culture in Ireland and the wider world*, edited by R.V. Comerford and Jennifer Kelly, pp. 179–90. Dublin: Irish Academic Press, 2010.

McKibbin, Ross. 'Great Britain'. In *Twisted paths: Europe, 1914–45*, edited by Robert Gerwarth, pp. 33–59. Oxford: Oxford University Press, 2007.

Miller, Kerby. 'Class, culture and immigrant group identity in the United States: The case of Irish-American ethnicity'. In *Immigration reconsidered: History, sociology and politics*, edited by Virginia Yans-McLaughlin, pp. 96–129. New York: Oxford University Press, 1990.

Milne, Ida. 'Influenza: The Irish Local Government Board's last great crisis'. In *Healthcare in Ireland and Britain from 1850*, edited by Donnacha Seán Lucey and Virginia Crossman, pp. 217–36. London: Institute of Historical Research, 2014.

O'Connor, Steven. 'Imperial continuities: Irish doctors and the British armed forces, 1922–45'. In *Medicine, health and Irish experiences of conflict, 1914–45*, edited by David Durnin and Ian Miller, pp. 191–205. Manchester: Manchester University Press, 2017.

O'Halpin, Eunan. 'Problematic killing during the war of independence and its aftermath: Civilian spies and informers'. In *Death and dying in Ireland, Britain and Europe: Historical perspectives*, edited by James Kelly and Mary Ann Lyons, pp. 317–48. Kildare: Irish Academic Press, 2013.

Orr, Phillip. '200,000 volunteer soldiers'. In *Our war: Ireland and the Great War*, edited by John Horne, pp. 63–94. Dublin: Royal Irish Academy, 2008.

O'Toole, Fintan. 'Beyond amnesia and piety'. In *Towards commemoration: Ireland in war and revolution 1912–23*, edited by John Horne and Edward Madigan, pp. 154–61. Dublin: Royal Irish Academy, 2013.

Panayi, Panikos. 'Anti-German riots in London during the First World War'. *German History* 7 (1989), pp. 184–203.

Pelis, Kim. 'Taking credit: The Canadian Army Medical Corps and the British conversion to blood transfusion in WW1'. *Journal of History of Medicine and Allied Sciences* 56 (2001), pp. 238–77.

Perry, Heather. 'Re-arming the disabled veteran'. In *Artificial parts, practical lives: Modern histories of prosthetics*, edited by Katherine Ott, David Serlin, and Stephen Mihm, pp. 75–101. New York: New York University Press, 2002.

Peterson, Jeanne. 'Gentlemen and medical men: The problem of professional recruitment'. *Bulletin of the History of Medicine* 58 (1984), pp. 457–73.

Rasmussen, Anne. 'The Spanish flu'. In *The Cambridge history of the First World War: Civil society*, edited by Jay Winter, pp. 334–57. Cambridge: Cambridge University Press, 2014.

Reznick, Jeffery. 'Work therapy and the disabled British soldier in Great Britain in the First World War: The case of Shepherd's Bush Military Hospital'. In *Disabled veterans in history*, edited by David A. Gerber, pp. 185–203. Ann Arbor, MI: The University of Michigan Press, 2000.

Riordan, Susannah. 'Venereal disease in the Irish free state: The politics of public health'. *Irish Historical Studies* 35, no. 139 (2007), pp. 345–64.

Robinson, Michael. '"Nobody's children?": The Ministry of pensions and the treatment of disabled Great War veterans in the Irish free state, 1921–1939'. *Irish Studies Review* 25, no. 3 (2017), pp. 316–35.

Staunton, Martin. 'Kilrush, Co. Clare and the Royal Munster Fusiliers: The experience of an Irishtown in the First World War'. *The Irish Sword* 16 (1986), pp. 268–72.

Supple, Barry. 'War economies'. In *The Cambridge history of the First World War: The state*, edited by Jay Winter, pp. 295–324. Cambridge: Cambridge University Press, 2014.

Van Bergen, Leo. '"The malingerers are to blame": The Dutch Military Health service before and during the First World War'. In *Medicine and modern warfare*, edited by Roger Cooter, Mark Harrison, and Steve Sturdy, pp. 59–76. Amsterdam: Clio Medica, 1999.

Van Bergen, Leo. 'Military medicine'. In *The Cambridge history of the First World War: Civil society*, edited by Jay Winter, pp. 287–309. Cambridge: Cambridge University Press, 2014.

Walsh, Fionnuala. '"Every human life is a national importance": The impact of the First World War on attitudes to maternal and infant health'. In *Medicine, health and Irish experiences of conflict, 1914–45*, edited by David Durnin and Ian Miller, pp. 15–30. Manchester: Manchester University Press, 2017.

Watson, Janet. 'A sister's war: The diaries of Alice Slythe'. In *First World War nursing: New perspectives*, edited by Alison S. Fell and Christine E. Hallett, pp. 103–22. London: Taylor & Francis, 2013.

Whitehead, Ian. 'The British Medical Officer on the Western Front: The training of doctors for war'. In *Medicine and modern warfare*, edited by Roger Cooter, Mark Harrison, and Steve Sturdy, pp. 163–84. Amsterdam: Clio Medica, 1999.

Winter, Jay. 'Hospitals'. In *Capital cities at war: Paris, London, Berlin, 1914–19: A cultural history*, edited by Jay Winter and Jean-Louis Robert, pp. 354–82. Cambridge: Cambridge University Press, 2012.

Wright, David, Mullally, Sasha, and Colleen Cordukes, Mary. 'Worse than being married: The exodus of British doctors from the National Health Service to Canada, *c*.1955–75'. *Journal of the History of Medicine and Allied Sciences* 65 (2010), pp. 546–75.

BOOKS

Abel-Smith, Brian. *The hospitals, 1800–1948*. London: Heinemann, 1964.

Ackroyd, Marcus, Brockliss, Laurence, Moss, Michael, Retford, Kate, and Stevenson, John. *Advancing with the army: Medicine, the professions and social mobility in the British Isles, 1790–1850*. Oxford: Oxford University Press, 2006.

Adams, Annmarie. *Medicine by design: The architect and the modern hospital, 1893–1943*. Minneapolis, MN: University of Minnesota Press, 2008.

Adams, Ralph, and Poirier, Phillip. *The conscription controversy in Great Britain, 1900–18*. Basingstoke: Macmillan, 1987.

Alter, Peter. *The reluctant patron: Science and the state in Britain, 1850–1920*. Oxford: Berg, 1987.

Barham, Peter. *Forgotten lunatics of the Great War*. London: Yale University Press, 2007.

Barrington, Ruth. *Health, medicine and politics in Ireland, 1900–70*. Dublin: Institute of Public Administration, 1987

Bew, Paul. *Ideology and the Irish question: Ulster unionism and Irish nationalism, 1912–16*. Oxford: Clarendon Press, 1994.

Blair, John. *Centenary history of the RAMC, 1898–1998*. Edinburgh: Iynx Publishing, 1998.

Bourke, Joanna. *Dismembering the male: Men's bodies, Britain and the Great War*. London: Reaktion, 1999.

Bourke, Joanna. *An intimate history of killing: Face to face killing in twentieth century warfare*. London: Granta Books, 1999.

Bowman, Timothy. *The Irish regiments in the Great War—Discipline and morale*. Manchester: Manchester University Press, 2003.

Boyce, David. *'The sure confusing drum': Ireland and the First World War*. Swansea: University College of Swansea, 1993.

Burke, Helen. *The Royal Hospital, Donnybrook: A heritage of caring, 1743–1993*. Dublin: Royal Hospital Donnybrook and the Social Science Research Centre, 1993.

Casey, P.J., Cullen, K.T., and Duignan, J.P. *Irish doctors in the First World War*. Kildare: Irish Academic Press, 2015.

Cassell, Ronald D. *Medical charities, medical politics: The Irish dispensary system and the poor law, 1836–1872*. Woodbridge: Royal Historical Society, 1997.

Coakley, Davis. *Doctor Steevens' Hospital.* Dublin: Dr. Steevens' Hospital Historical Centre, 1992.

Coakley, Davis. *Baggot Street: A short history of the Royal City of Dublin Hospital.* Dublin: Royal City of Dublin Hospital Governors, 1995.

Cohen, Susan. *Medical services in the First World War.* London: Bloomsbury, 2014.

Coleman, Marie. *The Irish sweep: A history of the Irish Hospitals sweepstake, 1930–87.* Dublin: University College Dublin Press, 2009.

Cooter, Roger. *Surgery and society in peace and war: Orthopaedics and the organization of modern medicine, 1880–1948.* London: Palgrave Macmillan, 1993.

Cox, Catherine. *Negotiating insanity in the southeast of Ireland, 1820–1900.* Manchester: Manchester University Press, 2012.

Crossman, Virginia. *Politics, pauperism and power in late nineteenth-century Ireland.* Manchester: Manchester University Press, 2006.

Crossman, Virginia. *Poverty and the poor law in Ireland, 1850–1914.* Liverpool: Liverpool University Press, 2013.

Crowther, M. Anne, and Dupree, Marguerite. *Medical lives in the age of surgical revolution.* Cambridge: Cambridge University Press, 2007.

Crozier, Anna. *Practising colonial medicine: The Colonial Medical Service in British East Africa.* London: I.B. Tauris, 2007.

Curtin, Phillip. *Death by migration: Europe's encounter with the tropical world in the nineteenth century.* Cambridge: Cambridge University Press, 1989.

Daly, Mary E. *Dublin the deposed capital: A social and economic history, 1860–1914.* Cork: Cork University Press, 1984.

Daly, Mary E. *The buffer state: The historical roots of the Department of the Environment.* Dublin: Institute of Public Administration, 1997.

Daly, Mary E. *The slow failure: Population decline and independent Ireland, 1920–73.* Madison, WI: University of Wisconsin Press, 2006.

Daly, Mary E. *The Irish state and the diaspora.* Dublin: National University of Ireland, 2008.

D'Arcy, Fergus. *Remembering the war dead: British Commonwealth and international war graves in Ireland since 1914.* Dublin: Stationary Office, 2007.

Delaney, Enda. *Demography, state and society: Irish migration to Britain, 1921–71.* Liverpool: Liverpool University Press, 2000.

Delaney, Enda. *Irish emigration since 1921.* Dublin: Economic and Social History Society of Ireland, 2002.

Delaney, Enda. *The Irish in post-war Britain.* Oxford: Oxford University Press, 2007.

Denman, Terrence. *Ireland's unknown soldiers: The 16th (Irish) division in the Great War, 1914–18.* Dublin: Irish Academic Press, 1992.

Digby, Anne. *Making a medical living: Doctors and patients in the English market for medicine, 1720–1911.* Cambridge: Cambridge University Press, 2002.

Dolan, Anne. *Commemorating the Irish Civil War: History and memory, 1923–2000.* Cambridge: Cambridge University Press, 2006.

Dooley, Thomas. *Irishmen or English soldiers?* Liverpool: Liverpool University Press, 1995.

Drew, Robert, and Peterkin, William. *Commissioned officers in the medical services of the British Army, 1660–1960.* London: Wellcome Historical Medical Library, 1968.

Duggan, John. *A history of the Irish Army.* Dublin: Gill and Macmillan, 1991.

Dungan, Myles. *They shall not grow old: Irish soldiers and the Great War.* Dublin: Four Courts Press, 1997.

Fealy, Gerard. *A history of apprenticeship nurse training in Ireland.* London: Routledge, 2005.

Ferriter, Diarmaid. *The transformation of Ireland, 1900–2000.* London: Profile Books, 2004.

Finnane, Mark. *Insanity and the insane in post-famine Ireland.* New York: ACLS History E-Book Project, 1981.

Fitzpatrick, David. *Irish emigration, 1801–1921.* Dublin: Economic and Social History Society of Ireland, 1984.

Fitzpatrick, David. *Ireland and the First World War.* Dublin: Lilliput Press, 1986.

Fitzpatrick, David. *Politics and Irish life 1913–21: Provincial experience of war and revolution.* Cork: Cork University Press, 1998.

Foley, Caitriona. *The last Irish plague: The great flu epidemic in Ireland, 1918–19.* Dublin: Irish Academic Press, 2011.

Freeman, E.T. *Mater Misericordiae Hospital: Centenary, 1861–1961.* Dublin: Mater Misericordiae Hospital, 1962.

Fussell, Paul. *The Great War and modern memory.* Oxford: Oxford University Press, 1975.

Gatenby, Peter. *Dublin's Meath Hospital, 1753–1996.* Dublin: Town House, 1996.

Geary, Laurence. *Medicine and charity in Ireland, 1718–1851.* Dublin: University College Dublin Press, 2004.

Gorsky, Martin, Mohan, John, and Willis, Tim. *Mutualism and health care: British hospital contributory schemes in the twentieth century.* Manchester: Manchester University Press, 2006.

Grayzel, Susan. *Women's identities at war: Gender, motherhood and politics in Britain and France during the First World War.* Chapel Hill: The University of North Carolina Press, 1999.

Gregory, Adrian. *The silence of memory, Armistice Day 1919–46.* Oxford: Berg, 1994.

Harrison, Mark. *The medical war: British military medicine in the First World War.* Oxford: Oxford University Press, 2010.

Hart, Peter. *The IRA and its enemies: Violence and community in Cork, 1916–23.* Oxford: Oxford University Press, 1998.

Hart, Peter. *The I.R.A. at war, 1916–23.* Oxford: Oxford University Press, 2003.

Hay, Ian. *One hundred years of army nursing: The story of the British Army nursing service from the time of Florence Nightingale to the present day.* London: Cassell, 1953.

Hennessy, Thomas. *Dividing Ireland: World War 1 and partition.* London: Routledge, 1998.

Honigsbaum, Frank. *The division in British medicine: A history of separation of general practice from hospital care, 1911–68.* London: Kogan Page, 1979.

Hopkinson, Michael. *Green against green: The Irish Civil War.* Dublin: Gill and Macmillan, 2004.

Hutchinson, John. *Champions of charity: War and the rise of the Red Cross.* Oxford: Westview, 1995.

Irish, Tomás. *Trinity in war and revolution, 1912–1923.* Dublin: Royal Irish Academy, 2015.

Jackson, Alvin. *Ireland, 1798–1998: Politics and war.* Oxford: Oxford University Press, 1999.

Jackson, Alvin. *Home rule: An Irish history, 1800–2000.* Oxford: Oxford University Press, 2003.

Jeffery, Keith. *Ireland and the Great War.* Cambridge: Cambridge University Press, 2000.

Johnstone, Tom. *Orange, green and khaki: The story of Irish regiments in the Great War.* Dublin: Gill and Macmillan, 1992.

Jones, Greta. '*Captain of all these men of death': The history of tuberculosis in nineteenth and twentieth century Ireland.* Amsterdam: Rodopi, 2001.

Kelly, Laura. *Irish women in medicine, c.1880s–1920s: Origins, education and careers.* Manchester: Manchester University Press, 2012.

Kelly, Laura. *Irish medical education and student culture, c.1850–1950.* Liverpool: Liverpool University Press, 2017.

Kissane, Bill. *The politics of the Irish War.* Oxford: Oxford University Press, 2005.

Kitchen, Martin. *Europe between the wars.* Harlow: Pearson Longman, 2006.

Laffan, Michael. *The partition of Ireland, 1911–1925.* Dundalk: Dundalgan Press, 1983.

Lee, Joseph J. *Ireland, 1912–1985: Politics and society.* Cambridge: Cambridge University Press, 1989.

Leed, Eric. *No man's land: Combat and identity in World War 1.* Cambridge: Cambridge University Press, 1979.

Leese, Peter. *Shell shock: Traumatic neurosis and the British soldiers of the First World War.* Basingstoke: Palgrave Macmillan, 2002.

Lerner, Paul. *Hysterical men: War psychiatry and the politics of trauma in Germany 1890–1930.* London: Cornell University Press, 2003.

Lovegrove, Peter. *Not least in the crusade: A short history of the Royal Army Medical Corps.* Aldershot: Gale & Polden, 1951.

Lucey, Donnacha Seán. *The end of the Irish Poor Law? Welfare and healthcare reform in revolutionary and independent Ireland*. Manchester: Manchester University Press, 2015.

Luddy, Maria. *Women in Ireland, 1800–1918*. Cork: Cork University Press, 1995.

Lyons, Martyn. *The writing culture of ordinary people in Europe, c.1860–1920*. Cambridge: Cambridge University Press, 2013.

MacKenzie, Simon. *Politics and military morale: Current affairs and citizenship education in the British Army, 1914–50*. Oxford: Clarendon Press, 1992.

McEwen, Yvonne. *It's a long way to Tipperary: British and Irish nurses during the Great War*. Dunfermline: Cualann Press, 2006.

McGann, Susan. *A history of the Royal College of Nursing, 1916–90*. Manchester: Manchester University Press, 2010.

McGarry, Fearghal. *The Rising: Easter 1916*. Oxford: Oxford University Press, 2010.

McIntosh, Gillian. *The force of culture: Unionist identities in twentieth-century Ireland*. Cork: Cork University Press, 1999.

McLaughlin, Redmond. *The Royal Army Medical Corps*. London: L Cooper, 1972.

Medical Missionaries of Mary. *A dream to follow: The story of Marie Helena Martin aged 23 to 33*. Dublin: Medical Missionaries of Mary, 2010.

Meenan, F.O.C. *Cecilia Street: The Catholic University School of Medicine, 1855–1931*. Dublin: Gill and Macmillan, 1987.

Meyer, Jessica. *Men of war: Masculinity and the First World War in Britain*. Basingstoke: Palgrave Macmillan, 2011.

Milne, Ida. *Stacking the coffins: Influenza, war and revolution in Ireland, 1918–19*. Manchester: Manchester University Press, 2018.

Mitchell, David. *'A peculiar place': The Adelaide Hospital, Dublin, 1839–1989*. Dublin: Blackwater Press, 1989.

Mitchell, Thomas, and Smith, G.M. *History of the Great War based on official documents: Casualties and medical statistics of the war*. London: HMSO, 1931.

Moloney, Senan. *Lusitania: An Irish tragedy*. Cork: Mercier, 2004.

Moore, Steven. *The Irish on the Somme*. Belfast: Local Press, 2005.

Mulligan, William. *The origins of the First World War*. Cambridge: Cambridge University Press, 2010.

Mulligan, William. *The Great War for peace*. New Haven: Yale University Press, 2014.

Murphy, Cliona. *The women's suffrage movement and Irish society in the early twentieth century*. Hemel Hempstead: Harvester Wheatsheaf, 1989.

Murphy, David. *Irish regiments in the world wars*. Oxford: Osprey, 2007.

Murphy, Oliver. *The cruel clouds of war*. Dublin: Belvedere Museum, 2003.

Murphy, William. *Political imprisonment and the Irish, 1912–21*. Oxford: Oxford University Press, 2014.

Novick, Ben. *Conceiving revolution: Irish nationalist propaganda during the First World War.* Dublin: Four Courts Press, 2001.

O'Connor, Steven. *Irish officers in the British forces, 1922–45.* Basingstoke: Palgrave Macmillan, 2014.

Oram, Gerard. *Worthless men: Race, eugenics and the death penalty in the British Army during the First World War.* London: Francis Boutle, 1998.

Orr, Phillip. *The road to the Somme: Men of the Ulster division tell their Story.* Belfast: Blackstaff Press, 1987.

Orr, Phillip. *Field of bones: An Irish division at Gallipoli.* Dublin: Lilliput Press, 2006.

Perkin, Harold. *The rise of professional society: England since 1880.* London: Routledge, 2016.

Purdon, Edward. *The Irish Civil War, 1922–23.* Cork: Mercier Press, 2000.

Rees, Peter. *'The other Anzacs': Nurses at war, 1914–18.* Crows Nest: Allen & Unwin, 2008.

Reynolds, Joseph. *Grangegorman: Psychiatric care in Dublin since 1815.* Dublin: Institute of Public Administration, 1992.

Richardson, Neil. *'A coward if I return, a hero if I fall': Stories of Irishmen in World War 1.* Dublin: O'Brien Press, 2010.

Ryan, Eugene P. *Haig's Medical Officer: The papers of Colonel Eugene 'Micky' Ryan.* Barnsley: Pen and Sword Military, 2013.

Seipp, Adam. *The ordeal of peace: Demobilization and the urban experience in Britain and Germany, 1917–21.* Surrey: Routledge, 2009.

Shephard, Ben. *A war of nerves: Soldiers and psychiatrists, 1914–44.* London: Pimlico, 2002.

Stevens, Rosemary. *Medical practice in modern England: The impact of specialization and state medicine.* New Haven: Yale University Press, 1971.

Stokes, Roy. *Death in the Irish sea: The sinking of the RMS Leinster.* Cork: Collins Press, 1998.

Taaffe, Michael. *Those days are gone away.* London: Hutchinson, 1959.

Taylor, James. *The 1st Royal Irish Rifles in the Great War.* Dublin: Four Courts Press, 2002.

Taylor, James. *The 2nd Royal Irish Rifles in the First World War.* Dublin: Four Courts Press, 2005.

Taylor, Paul. *Heroes or traitors? Experiences of Southern Irish soldiers returning from the Great War, 1919–1939.* Liverpool: Liverpool University Press, 2015.

Townsend, Charles. *Easter 1916: The Irish Rebellion.* London: Penguin Books, 2006.

Tyquin, Michael. *Gallipoli: The medical war. The Australian Army Medical Services in the Dardanelles campaign of 1915.* Kensington: NSW University Press, 1993.

Van Bergen, Leo. *Before my helpless sight: Suffering, dying and military medicine on the Western Front, 1914–1918.* Surrey: Routledge, 2009.

Vaughan, W.E., and Fitzpatrick, A.J. *Irish historical statistics, population, 1821–1971*. Dublin: Royal Irish Academy, 1978.

Whalen, Robert. *Bitter wounds: German victims of the Great War, 1914–39*. London: Cornell University Press, 1984.

Whitehead, Ian. *Doctors in the Great War*. Barnsley: Pen and Sword, 1999.

Widdess, J.D.H. *The charitable infirmary, Jervis Street, 1718–1968*. Dublin: Jervis Street, 1968.

Widdess, J.D.H. *The Richmond, Whitworth and Hardwicke Hospitals, St Laurence's Dublin, 1772–1972*. Dublin: House of Industry Hospitals, 1972.

Willoughby, Roger. *A military history of the University of Dublin and its Officer Training Corps, 1910–22*. Limerick: Medal Society of Ireland, 1989.

Winter, Denis. *Death's men: Soldiers of the Great War*. London: Penguin Books, 2014.

Winter, Jay. *The Great War and the British people*. London: Macmillan, 1985.

Yeates, Padraig. *A city in wartime: Dublin 1914–18*. Dublin: Gill and Macmillan, 2012.

UNPUBLISHED THESES

Brennan, John Martin. 'Irish Catholic Chaplains in the First World War' (MPhil thesis, University of Birmingham, 2012).

Callan, Patrick. 'Voluntary recruiting for the British Army in Ireland during the First World War' (PhD thesis, University College, Dublin, 1984).

O'Neill, Clare. 'The Irish Home Front 1914–18 with particular reference to the treatment of Belgian refugees, prisoners-of-war, enemy Aliens and war casualties' (PhD thesis, Maynooth University, 2006).

# INDEX

© The Editor(s) (if applicable) and The Author(s),
under exclusive license to Springer Nature Switzerland AG 2019
D. Durnin, *The Irish Medical Profession and the First World War*,
Medicine and Biomedical Sciences in Modern History,
https://doi.org/10.1007/978-3-030-17959-5

The manufacturer's authorised representative in the EU is Springer
Nature Customer Service Centre GmbH, Europaplatz 3, 69115 Heidelberg,
Germany. If you have any concerns regarding our products, please
contact ProductSafety@springernature.com

Printed and bound by CPI Group (UK) Ltd, Croydon, CR0 4YY
29/04/2026
02099478-0009